Smoothies

D1742180

This Book Includes:

Green Smoothies &

Vegan Protein Smoothies

By Karen Greenvang

Copyright ©Karen Greenvang 2016

All rights reserved. No part of this publication may be reproduced, stored in a retrieval system, or transmitted, in any form or by any means, electronic, mechanical, photocopying, recording or otherwise, without the prior written permission of the author and the publishers.

The scanning, uploading, and distribution of this book via the Internet, or via any other means, without the permission of the author is illegal and punishable by law. Please purchase only authorized electronic editions, and do not participate in or encourage electronic piracy of copyrighted materials.

All information in this book has been carefully researched and checked for factual accuracy. However, the author and publishers make no warranty, expressed or implied, that the information contained herein is appropriate for every individual, situation or purpose, and assume no responsibility for errors or omission. The reader assumes the risk and full responsibility for all actions, and the author will not be held liable for any loss or damage, whether consequential, incidental, and special or otherwise, that may result from the information presented in this publication.

All cooking is an experiment in a sense, and many people come to the same or similar recipe over time. All recipes in this book have been derived from author's personal experience. Should any bear a close resemblance to those used elsewhere, that is purely coincidental.

The book is not intended to provide medical advice or to take the place of medical advice and treatment from your personal physician. Readers are advised to consult their own doctors or other qualified health professionals regarding the treatment of medical conditions. The author shall not be held liable or responsible for any misunderstanding or misuse of the information contained in this book. The information is not intended to diagnose, treat or cure any disease.

It is important to remember that the author of this book is not a doctor/ medical professional. Only opinions based upon her own personal experiences or research are cited. **THE AUTHOR DOES NOT OFFER MEDICAL ADVICE or prescribe any treatments. For any health or medical issues – you should be talking to your doctor first.**

Table of Contents

Book 1

Book 1
Green Smoothies

Alkaline Green Smoothie Recipes to Detox, Lose Weight, and Feel Energized

By Karen Greenvang

Copyright ©Karen Greenvang 2016

Introduction

Green Smoothies have come front and center for a meal choice, snack, or even a dessert. Holistic foods, green leafy vegetables, and proper hydration are hailed in supporting a healthy immune system, excellent energy, and helping ensure longevity. Green smoothies are a part of supporting all three. Best of all green smoothies are delicious and different. They offer an easy alternative to chopping up all the vegetables for a salad. If you drink green smoothies, your energy will increase, your skin will look better, and most of all you feel good. There are so many different food choices to put in green smoothies, and this book uses the plethora of natural healthy foods to make new and interesting green smoothie recipes.

The recipes in this book are full of exciting ingredients. Foods like Spirulina, chia seeds, almond milk, cashew milk, and more. The combinations are endless for making vegan green smoothies, especially with all the great options in the health food stores, and the health food section in regular conventional grocery stores.

The recipes in this book have been especially created for excellent taste and the content of ingredients for your health. None of these green smoothie recipes have dairy or honey in them. The sweetness of these smoothies comes naturally from fruit, and sweet vegetables such as carrots and beets, and other foods that add flavor and texture to the smoothies.

The point of a green smoothie is to get your dose of leafy green vegetables. The smoothies in this book may look one way and taste another. The best thing you can do is make all the smoothies and find the ones that you like the best. There are smoothies in this book that are green and taste more like veggies, and there smoothie recipes where the drink may be green yet taste more like a creamy milk shake. You probably have different tastes at different times. These recipes provide you with these different flavors to satisfy your food cravings in a healthy way.

I congratulate you for choosing to be healthy. Choosing to make a smoothie for a snack or a meal is beneficial to your health and mind. You will be strengthening your bones, muscles, and helping your energy level by making and drinking these smoothies every day, along with healthy exercise you are taking care of yourself. I hope you enjoy the recipes, and now let's take a look at some green smoothie recipes!

This book is not only for vegans or plant-based diet followers. Everyone can benefit from adding more fresh fruits and vegetables into their diet and green smoothies are great for that. If you are not a vegan, but would like to eat more vegan/plant-based, this book will show you how. Everyone is welcome here!

This is going to be an incredibly healthy, holistic journey that will help you explore the green, raw-vegan world. If you would like to improve your health, I suggest you start with a very simple goal- try to have just one green smoothie a day and take it from there. I am not suggesting you should go on a drastic, unrealistic cleanse (all kinds of cleanses and drastic changes to your diet should always be discussed with a medical professional first); all you should focus on is adding. Adding what? More superfood green smoothies. Yummy!

Before we dive into the recipes, I would like to offer you a free, complimentary recipe eBook with delicious vegan superfood smoothies.

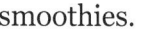

Download it now, before you forget.

www.bitly.com/karenfreegift

If you have any problems with your download, email me at: karenveganbooks@gmail.com

The Recipes

Recipe Measurements

I love keeping ingredient measurements as simple as possible- this is why I stick to tablespoons, teaspoons and cups.

The cup measurement I use is the American cup measurement. I also use it for dry ingredients. If you are new to it, let me help you:

If you don't have American Cup measures, just use a metric or imperial liquid measuring jug and fill your jug with your ingredient to the corresponding level. Here's how to go about it:

1 American Cup= 250ml= 8 fl.oz

For example:

If a recipe calls for 1 cup of almonds, simply place your almonds into your measuring jug until it reaches the 250 ml/8oz mark.

I know that different countries use different measurements and I wanted to make things simple for you.

Kale and Cashew Smoothie

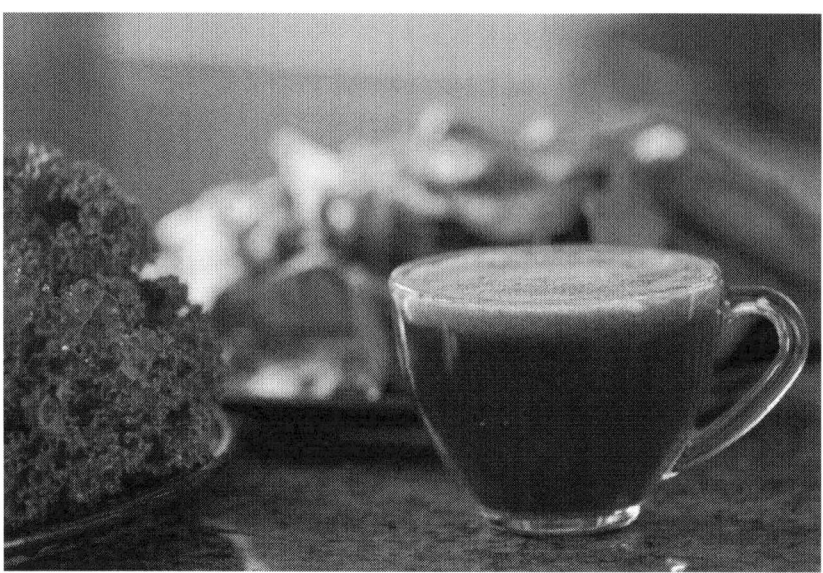

Serves 1-2

Ingredients

- 3/4 cup of fresh Pineapple
- 1 cup Cold Unsweetened Cashew Milk
- 1 cup of Kale
- 2 drops of Chlorophyll
- ½ cup of crushed ice

Directions

1. Cut the leaves off the top of the pineapple.
2. Cut the spikey skin from the pineapple.
3. Cut the pineapple in four sections by cutting the meat away from the core.
4. Cut up pineapple meat and measure ¾ of a cup of pineapple.
5. Put the crushed ice into the blender and pour in the cold unsweetened cashew milk.
6. Wash the kale.

7. Pull kale leaves away from the stems.
8. Put the kale into the blender along with the chlorophyll. Place the top on the blender and blend on low until everything is mixed.
9. The crushed ice is optional if you would a creamier smoothie. You can taste and add more milk or pineapple if need be. Pour into a glass and garnish with a piece of pineapple on the rim and a straw. Smoothies can be much easier to drink with a straw.

Cabbage Coconut Chia Smoothie

Serves 1-2

Ingredients

- 1/2 cup of cabbage
- 1 cup cold unsweetened coconut milk
- 1 tablespoon of chia seeds
- 1/2 cup of cherries
- 1/2 cup of spinach

Directions

1. Pour the coconut milk into the blender.
2. Cut up the cabbage and put in the blender.
3. Place chia seeds in a coffee grinder and chop to a powder. Brush the powder into the blender.
4. Make sure the cherries do not have pits in them.
5. Place the pit less cherries into the mix.
6. Wash and dry the spinach.
7. Chop up fresh spinach and put in the mix, with the cover on the blender mix on low and them medium.
8. Press puree for a bit and make sure all foods are well blended and copped up.
9. The more you chop up a vegetable before it goes in the blender, the better the mix will be.
10. Taste the blend and see if you like the texture and the flavor. You can gradually add more of any of the ingredients to change the smoothie a little bit. Pour into a glass and enjoy.

Banana Broccoli Smoothie

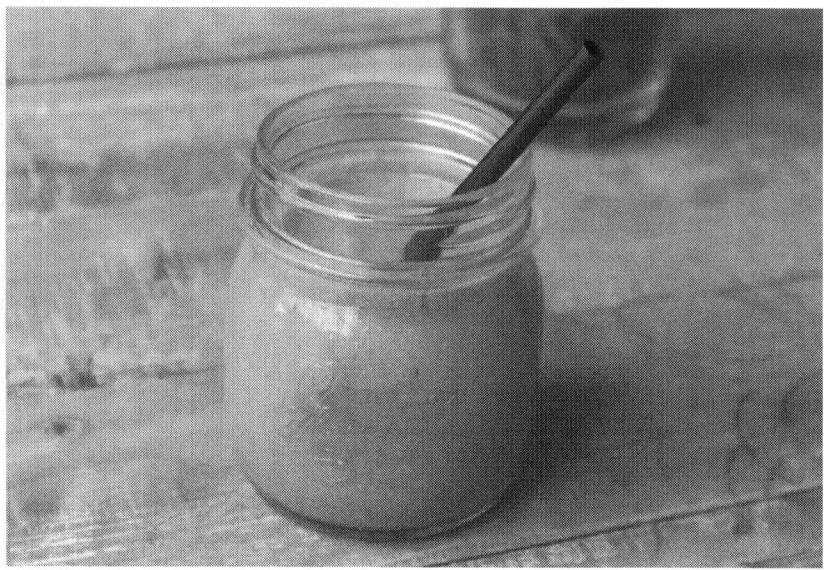

Serves: 1-2

Ingredients:

- 1 1/2 peeled frozen bananas
- 1 cup almond milk
- ½ cup of cooked broccoli
- ½ cup of kale leaves

Directions

1. Place the peeled bananas in the freezer overnight.
2. In the cut up the bananas and put in blender with the almond milk.
3. Cook broccoli and put in the one half of a cup.
4. You can cook the kale or just put in the raw kale leaves.
5. Wash the kale before use.
6. Make sure to take the leaves off the cores.
7. Throw the cores away.
8. Blend all the ingredients on low until mixed.
9. Then mix ingredient on medium or if there is a puree button.

10. You want everything to reduce down to a smooth consistency.
11. If you need more smooth just add either more almond or a little water is always good as well.
12. Taste the smoothie and add more of any the ingredients if you need to for a slightly different taste.
13. Once you like the smoothie, pour in a glass and serve the smoothie with a straw.

Apple Carrot Kale Smoothie

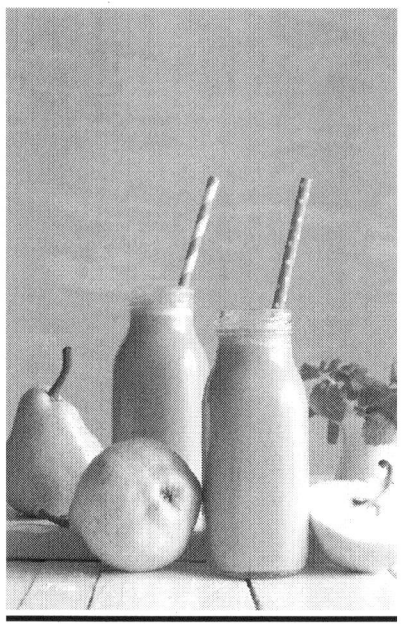

Serves 1-2

Ingredients

- 1 apple of your choice
- ½ cup of carrot juice
- ¾ cup of kale
- 1 teaspoon of fresh ginger

Directions

1. If you have a juicer, juice the apple and ½ cup of carrots and ginger.
2. If you do not have a juicer then buy apple juice that is 100 % apple juice and no sugar added.
3. The same for the carrot juice.
4. You can buy a container of 100 % carrot juice to do the job.
5. Make sure there is no sugar added.
6. Wash and dry the kale.

7. Pull the leaves away from the cores of the kale.
8. If you do not have a juicer then peel away the outside of the ginger.
9. Add the ginger into mix with all other ingredients.
10. Add the kale to the blender mix and mix on medium.
11. Increase the speed in order to make sure the kale blends up as much as possible.
12. The puree button should help to chop up smaller pieces.
13. All blenders are different.
14. Once the smoothie is blended, taste and add more of any of the ingredients gradually to change the flavor.
15. Once you have a taste you like pour the smoothie into a nice glass and enjoy with a drinking straw.

Spirulina Mango Coconut Smoothie

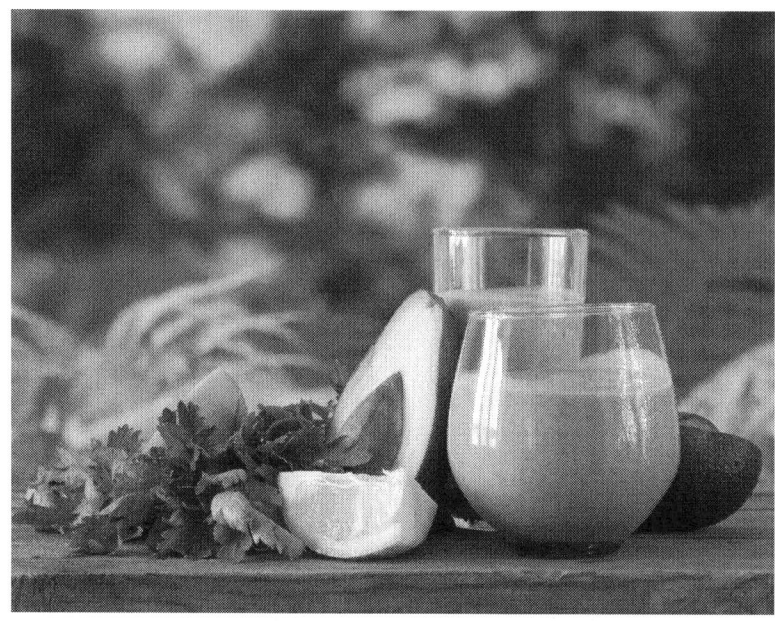

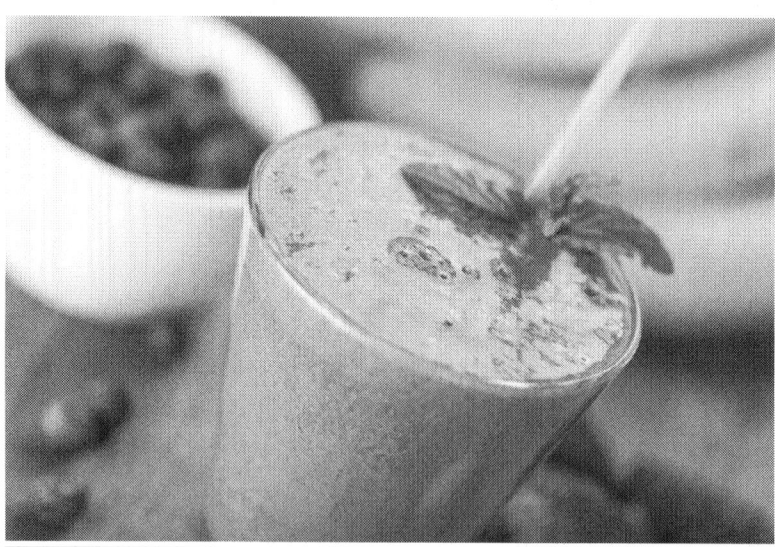

Serves 1-2

Ingredients

- 1 teaspoon of Spirulina
- 1 cup of frozen mango
- 1 cup of unsweetened coconut milk
- ½ cup spinach

Directions

1. Cut up the mango the night before.
2. Make sure you peel the skin off of the mango and take out the pit.
3. You want to get the pinkest mango you can for it to be ripe.
4. Put the mango bits in the freezer overnight in a container.
5. In the morning add your frozen mango, cup of unsweetened coconut milk, teaspoon of Spirulina, and spinach to the blender.
6. Put the blender on low to medium and blend until smooth.
7. When smoothie is well blended check the taste, adjust if you need to.
8. When you have the desired taste pour the smoothie in a glass and serve.

Avocado Blueberry Cherry Smoothie

Serves 1-2

Ingredients

- 1 Avocado soft to the touch
- ¾ cup of fresh then frozen blueberries
- ½ cup of pitted fresh cherries then frozen
- ½ teaspoon lemon
- ½ cup of 100 % no sugar added apple juice

Directions

1. Cut the avocado in half and twist one half avocado gently off of the pit.
2. Spoon the avocado meat into the blender.
3. Pour the apple juice and lemon juice into the blender.
4. Add the cherries and the blueberries to the blender.
5. Blend the mix on low to medium, mixing everything thoroughly.
6. Taste the smoothie and see if you need to add any of the ingredients for taste.
7. When you are ready pour the smoothie into a glass serve with a straw with a straw.

Cocoa Kale Almond Smoothie

Serves 1-2

Ingredients

- 1 tablespoon cocoa powder
- 1 frozen banana
- ½ cup almond milk
- 2 dates
- ½ cup of kale or cabbage

Directions

1. Put the banana in the freezer the night before you will make the smoothie.
2. Peel it first and then put it in a freezer appropriate container.
3. Pour the almond milk into the blender.
4. Pull the leaves of kale away from the stems and cut the kale as small as possible.
5. Put the cut up kale in the blender.
6. Cut the dates in half and take out the pit.
7. Cut the banana in thirds and put in the mix.
8. Blend ingredients together on low to medium.
9. Make sure everything is mixed together, well.
10. Pour into a glass and serve with a straw.

Orange Coconut Maca Smoothie

Serves 1-2

Ingredients

- 1 sweet large orange
- 1 cup of unsweetened coconut milk
- 1 frozen banana
- 1 tablespoon Maca powder

Directions

1. Peel the large orange and cut into four sections.
2. If your orange has seeds in it make sure you that you take the seeds out.
3. You can juice the orange and then throw the remaining seedless pulp into the bender. Just make sure you do not get any seeds in the blender.
4. Pour the coconut milk in the blender along with the cut up frozen banana and Maca powder.
5. Blend everything on low to medium until well blended.
6. Taste a bit to see if you like it and add more of any of the ingredients to change the flavor a bit.
7. When you have the desired taste pour smoothie into a glass and serve with a straw.

Barley Grass Lime Smoothie

Serves 1-2

Ingredients

- 1 to 2 teaspoons of barley grass powder
- ½ cup of frozen raspberries
- ½ cup frozen blueberries
- 1 lime
- ½ cup of apple juice

Directions

1. Pour the apple juice into the blender.
2. Add the frozen raspberries and blueberries to the blender.
3. Squeeze the lime until you have one tablespoon.
4. Put the juice of the lime into the blender.
5. Blend together all the ingredients until they are smooth.
6. Taste the smoothie and see if you like it. If you need to add a little more of the ingredients to suit your taste, do so.
7. When you have the desired taste, cut a ½ inch slice of lime.
8. Cut a slit into the lime and put it on the rim of the glass for garnish.
9. Serve in a glass with a straw.

Chia Milk Beet Smoothie

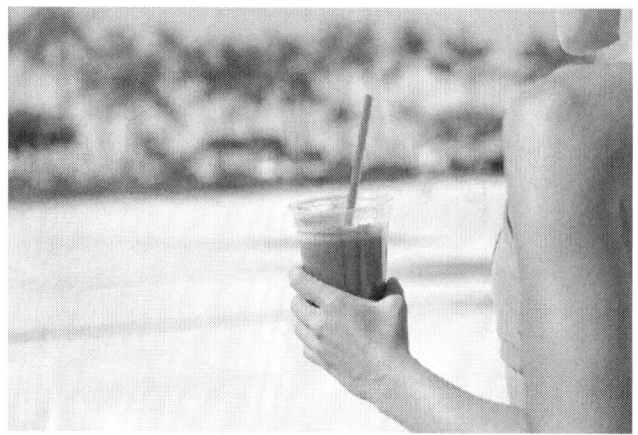

Serves 1-2

Ingredients

- 2 tablespoons chia seeds
- 2 ¼ cup of water
- ½ teaspoon vanilla
- 1 tablespoon agave syrup
- 3 tablespoons coconut pulp
- ½ cup of beets
- ½ cup collard greens
- 1 peeled pear

Directions

1. In a coffee grinder or blender make powder out of the chia seeds.
2. The coffee grinder works best.
3. Mix together chia seed powder and the water together in a blender on medium speed. Then add the agave, coconut pulp, and vanilla.
4. Mix everything together in the blender on medium speed.
5. Pour into a glass or bowl and let sit in the refrigerator overnight.

6. In the morning or whenever you are ready to make your smoothie pour 1 cup of chia seed milk and the beets into the blender.
7. Mix the ingredients on low to medium until they are mixed.
8. Then add the collard greens and the peeled pear.
9. Make sure you take the seeds and core out of the pear.
10. Only use the white pear meat.
11. Mix everything on low to medium in the blender.
12. When the ingredients are fully mixed taste the smoothie and if you need to add some more of any of the ingredients go ahead and do so.
13. When you have your desired taste pour the smoothie in a glass and serve with a straw.

Apricot and Cashew Green Smoothie

Serves 1-2

Ingredients

- ¾ cup of fresh, dried or canned apricots
- 1 banana
- ¾ cup of cashew milk
- 2 teaspoons chlorophyll
- 1/4 cup of peas
- 1 date

Directions

1. Put a peeled banana cut in half in the freezer overnight in a container.
2. The next morning cook the peas if they are frozen.
3. If you are using canned peas then you will just put them into the blender.
4. Add the cashew milk, chlorophyll, frozen banana halves, and apricots.
5. Mix in the blender on low to medium until the ingredients are thoroughly mixed.
6. Cut the pit out of the date and put in the blender.
7. Blend the mix on low to medium until everything is smooth and mixed.
8. Taste the smoothie and one or more of the ingredients a little at a time until you get your desired taste.
9. When you like what you taste then pour the smoothie in a glass and serve with a straw.

Papaya Cherry Smoothie

Serves 1-2

Ingredients

- ½ fresh papaya
- ½ cup coconut milk
- 1 teaspoon Spirulina
- ½ cup of cherries
- 1 date

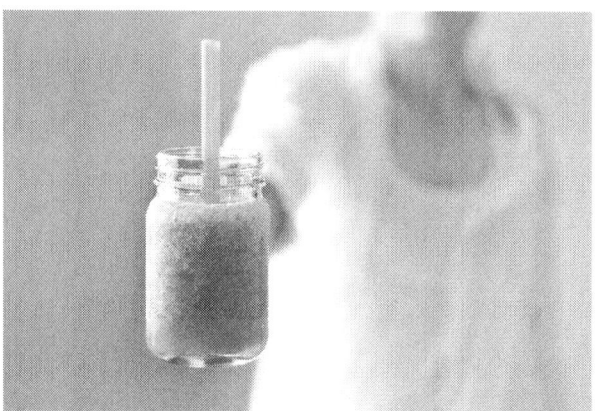

Directions

1. Cut the fresh papaya in half.
2. Take the brown seeds out with a spoon.
3. Cut the green-yellow skin from the outside of the papaya.
4. Cut up the papaya meat from half of the papaya and put it in the blender.
5. Pour the coconut milk into the blender.
6. Spoon the Spirulina in to the mix.
7. Cut up the cherries and take the pits out.
8. Put cherries into the mix.
9. Take the pit out of the date.
10. Put the date meat into the mix.

11. Blend the ingredients in the blender on a low to medium speed.
12. Blend until the mix is blended well.
13. Taste and make sure the smoothie has your desired taste.
14. You can gradually add a little more of one or more of the ingredients to get the taste you desire.
15. When you like the taste of the smoothie serve the smoothie in a nice glass along with a drinking straw.

Watermelon Smoothie

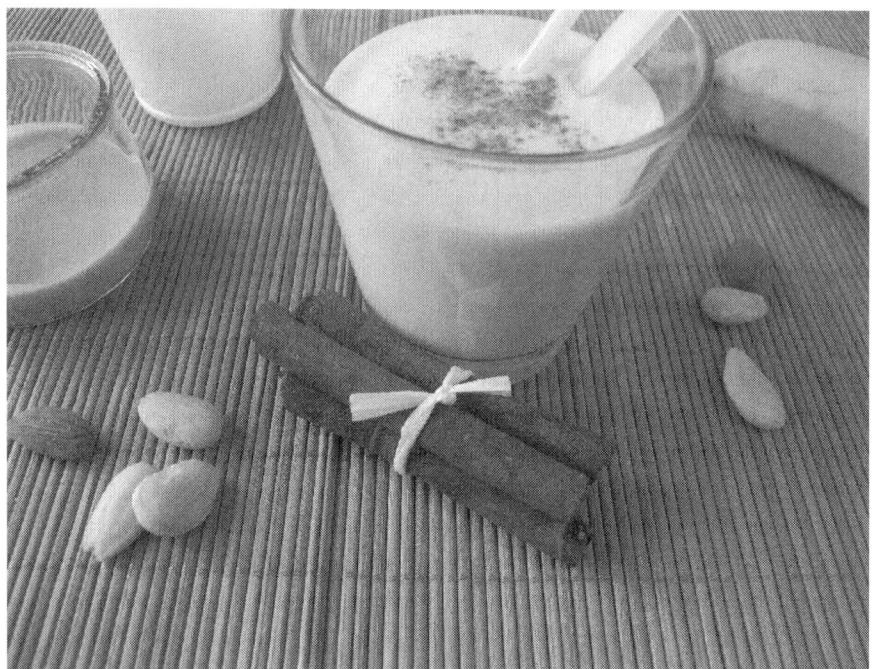

Serves 1-2

Ingredients

- 1 cup of water melon
- ¾ cup of blue berries
- 1 banana
- ½ cup of kale
- 1 teaspoon barley grass
- ½ broccoli

Directions

1. Peel the banana the night before you want to make the smoothie.
2. Put the cut banana in the freezer overnight.
3. Cut the rind off the watermelon and make sure you take the seeds out as well.

4. Cut the water melon into cubes.
5. Put the watermelon in the blender.
6. Add the blueberries and barley grass to the blender.
7. Pull the leaves off the stems of the kale.
8. Add the banana and the kale to the mixture.
9. The broccoli can be put into the blender raw, but it sometimes tastes better if you cook the broccoli first.
10. You can try the smoothies both ways and decide which one you like.
11. Cut the broccoli away from any big stems.
12. But up the broccoli and throw it into boiling water.
13. Let it simmer for no more than five minutes.
14. Cook the broccoli just until it is soft.
15. This allows for the most amount of nutrients to stay in the broccoli.
16. Put the broccoli raw or cooked in the blender with the rest of the ingredients and blend together on low to medium.
17. When the mixture is blended well, serve in a glass with a straw.

Honeydew Chia Berry Smoothie

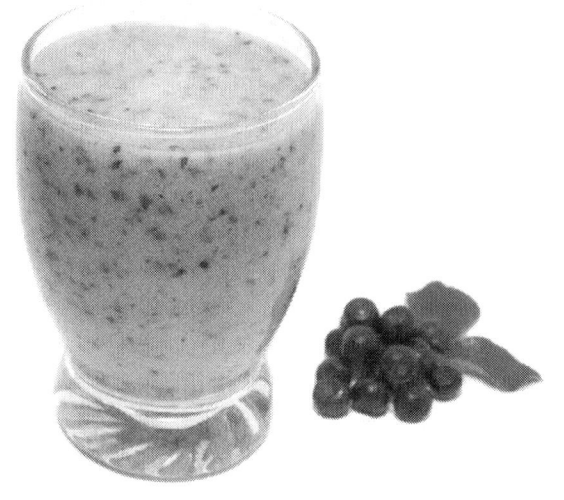

Serves 1-2

Ingredients

- 1 cup honeydew melon
- 1 date
- ½ cup of apple juice
- ½ fresh then frozen raspberries
- ½ cup of spinach
- ½ chia seed powder
- 1 teaspoon lemon

Directions

1. Put the fresh raspberries in a freezer appropriate container and place the container in the freezer the night before.
2. When you are ready to make the smoothie take the raspberries out of the freezer.

26

3. Cut up the honeydew melon and make sure to cut the hard skin from the honeydew melon.
4. Spoon out the seeds before measuring the melon into a cup.
5. Cut the pit out of the date.
6. Pour the ½ cup of apple juice into the blender.
7. Put the date and the honeydew melon into the blender.
8. Then put the frozen raspberries and lemon juice into the blender.
9. Make the chia seed powder in a coffee grinder by grinding the chia seeds.
10. Measure out the spinach leaves and put the spinach and the chia seed powder into the blender.
11. Blend all the ingredients on low to medium.
12. Make sure everything is blended well.
13. Taste to make sure you like.
14. Gradually add more of one or more ingredients if you need to.
15. Pour smoothie in a glass with a straw.

Very Berry Smoothie

Serves 1-2

Ingredients

- 1 cup of fresh then frozen raspberries
- ½ cup of fresh then frozen strawberries
- 2 teaspoons chlorophyll
- 1 cup of cold coconut milk
- ½ cup of kale
- ½ cup of blueberries

Directions

1. Wash the strawberries and raspberries and place them into the freezer overnight.
2. In the morning pour the cold coconut milk into the blender.
3. Take the kale leaves off of the stems.
4. Add the chlorophyll, kale, and blueberries to the blender.
5. Blend all the ingredients together on low to medium speed.
6. Make sure that all ingredients are well blended.
7. Taste and make sure you like the smoothie.
8. If you need to gradually add one or more of the ingredients to the taste.
9. When you are ready pour the smoothie into a glass and serve with a straw.

Pear Smoothie

Server 1-2

Ingredients

- 2 pears
- 1 teaspoon cinnamon
- ½ cup of cashew milk
- ½ cup of apple juice
- ½ cup of melon

Directions

1. Take the two pears wash them and cut the skins off of the outside of the pears.
2. Cut the pears in half and cut the pear meat away from the core of the pear.
3. Put the pear meat into the blender.
4. Measure the ½ teaspoon of cinnamon and put into the blender.
5. Add the cashew milk, apple juice, and melon.
6. Mix all the ingredients together on a low to medium speed.
7. Mix until the ingredients are well blended.
8. Taste your smoothie and gradually add a small amount of ingredients if need.
9. When you like the taste of the smoothie pour the smoothie into a glass with a straw and serve.

Ginger Smoothie

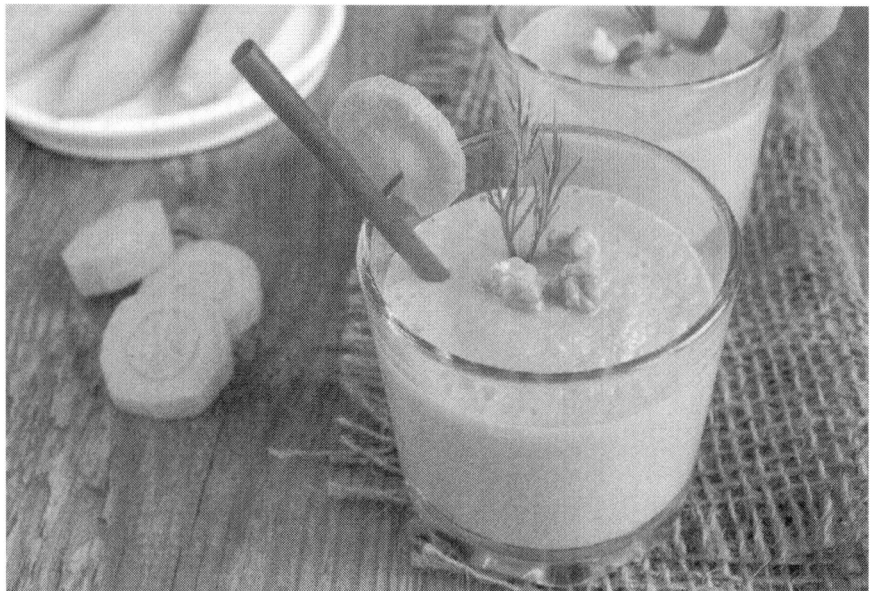

Serves 1-2

Ingredients

- 2 teaspoons ginger
- 2 dates
- ½ cup of kale
- ½ cup of apple juice
- Juice of half of a lemon

Directions

1. Take the ginger and cut the skin from the outside.
2. Take the dates and cut the pit from the center of the dates.
3. Put the ginger and dates into the blender.
4. Pull the kale leaves away from the core.
5. Put the kale in the blender and pour in the apple juice as well.

6. Squeeze the juice of the lemon into a glass and make sure to take out all of the seeds. Then pour the lemon into the blender.
7. Mix all the ingredients in the blender on a low to medium speed.
8. Make sure everything is blended well and copped up as much as possible.
9. Taste and adjust for desired taste if you need to.
10. Pour the smoothie into a glass and serve with a straw.

Cocoa Mint Smoothie

Serves 1-2

Ingredients

- ¼ cup of fresh mint
- ½ cup of cold almond milk
- 1 tablespoon of cocoa powder
- 1 banana

Directions

1. Peel the banana and cut it in half.
2. Put the banana in the freezer in a freezer appropriate container the night before making the smoothie.
3. Wash the mint and cut the mint as small as you can.
4. Pour the almond milk in the blender.
5. Put the mint, the tablespoon of cocoa powder, and the frozen banana in the blender. Blend on low to medium until all the ingredients are as small as they can be and everything is blended well.
6. Taste and adjust if you need to.
7. Pour the smoothie into a glass and drink with a straw.

Chamomile Kale Smoothie

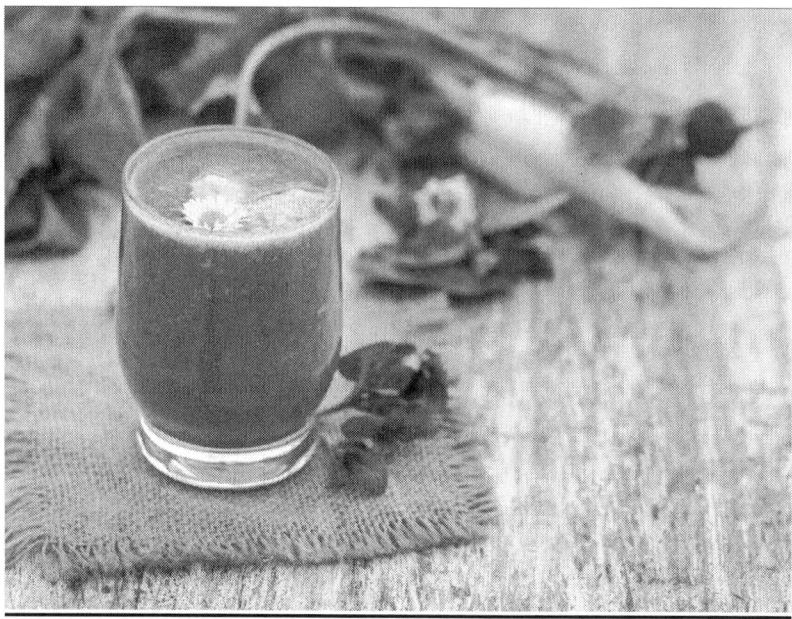

Serves 1-2

Ingredients

- 1 cup of chamomile tea
- ½ cup of almond milk
- ½ banana
- ½ cup of kale
- 2 date
- ½ cup of brewer's yeast

Directions

1. Buy a strong healthy good quality chamomile tea.
2. Make a cup and put two tea bags in so that the chamomile gets a nice and strong flavor. Put the chamomile tea in the refrigerator so it cools before you make the smoothie.
3. You can make the tea the night before.

4. When it is time to make the smoothie pour the almond milk in the blender.
5. Peel the banana and add it to the blend.
6. Pull the kale leaves away from the stems and add ½ cup of kale to the mix.
7. Cut the dates in half and remove the pits.
8. Put the brewer's yeast and dates into the blender.
9. Mix all the ingredients in the blender until they are all well mixed.
10. All the ingredients should be in the smallest form possible.
11. Taste and adjust smoothie by gradually adding one or more ingredients if you need to.
12. When the smoothie is ready pour it into a glass and serve smoothie with a straw.

Olive Oil Green Smoothie

Serves 1-2

Ingredients

- 1 tablespoon olive oil
- ½ cup of apple juice
- ½ cup of broccoli
- ½ cup of artichokes
- ½ cup of kale
- ½ cup of arugula
- 1 pear
- Dash of salt

Directions

1. Cook the broccoli so it is soft.
2. Buy artichokes in a glass container.
3. Add olive oil, apple juice, broccoli, and artichokes to the blender and mix on low to medium.
4. Then pull the kale leaves from the kale stems.
5. Cut the pear in half and peel away the skin.
6. Then cut away the core and stem.
7. Put pear meat and the kale into the blender and mix on low to medium.
8. Put the dash of salt in with the ingredients.
9. Mix all the ingredients until they are all in small pieces and the liquid is smooth to drink. Taste and adjust if you need to. When the smoothie is ready pour the smoothie into a glass with a straw.

Lavender Strawberry Smoothie

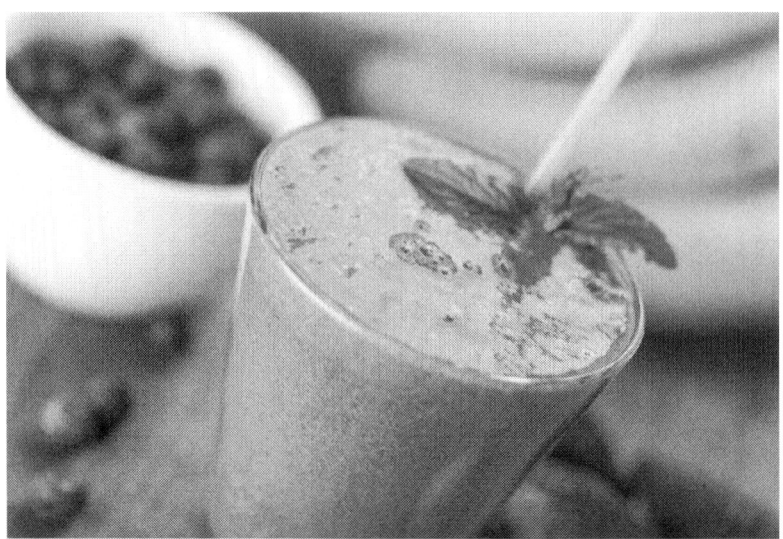

Serves 1-2

Ingredients

- 1 teaspoon of culinary lavender
- 2 cups of water
- 2 sprigs of mint
- ½ cucumber
- ½ cup of Strawberries
- 1 teaspoon Spirulina

Directions

1. In a large glass jug add the teaspoon of culinary lavender and the 2 cups of water.
2. Put the two sprigs of mint into the jug.
3. Put in the refrigerator for two hours and take out the sprig of mint.
4. Then keep the lavender mixture in the refrigerator for three more hours.
5. Then strain the lavender from the water.

6. Add lavender water to the blender.
7. Peel the cucumber and measure out ½ cup of cucumber meat and put it in the blender. Cut the green leaves off of the strawberries.
8. Also add the strawberries and Spirulina to the blender.
9. Mix all the ingredients together until smooth and well blended.
10. Taste and adjust if you need to.
11. Serve the smoothie in a glass cold with a straw to drink.

Vanilla Smoothie

Seres 1-2

Ingredients

- 1 natural vanilla bean
- ½ cup of cashew milk
- ½ banana
- 2 tablespoons brewer's yeast
- ½ cup of kale

Directions

1. Take the vanilla bean and press it flat with your fingers.
2. Then take a knife and gently split the vanilla bean open and scoop out the fresh vanilla specs with a spoon.
3. Pour the cashew milk into the blender.
4. Peel the banana and put the banana into the blender.
5. Then put the vanilla and the brewer's yeast in the mix.
6. Also separate the kale leaves from the stems and add the kale to the blender as well. Turn the speed on low and gradually use medium in order to blend all the ingredients together.
7. Blend the mix well so everything is pureed. When smoothie is at desired flavor, pour the smoothie into a glass and serve with a straw.

Cinnamon Smoothie

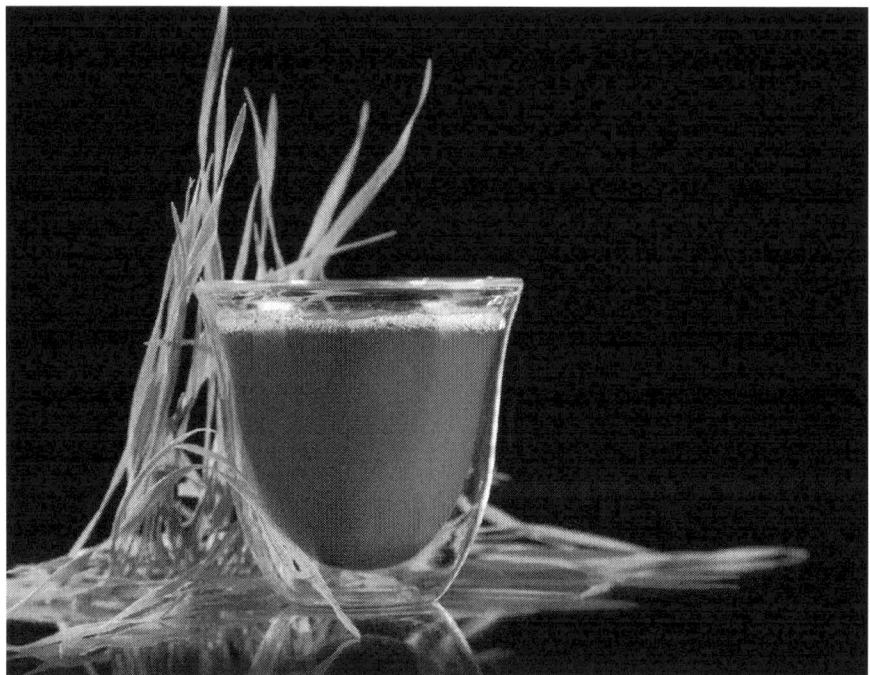

Serves 1-2

Ingredients

- 2 teaspoons of cinnamon
- ½ cup of almond milk
- 1 apple
- ½ cup of broccoli
- 1 teaspoon barley grass

Directions

1. Cook the broccoli just until it is soft.
2. Pour the almond milk in the blender.
3. Add the ingredients of cinnamon and broccoli along with the barley grass.

4. You can buy fresh cinnamon sticks and grate the cinnamon sticks with a grater until you have enough to fill two teaspoons.
5. Take the peel off of the apple and remove the seed, stem, if it has one, and the core.
6. Put the apple meat into the blender.
7. Turn the blender speed to low and gradually raise to medium.
8. Mix all of the ingredients together until well blended.
9. Taste your smoothie and adjust if you need to by adding a small amount of one or more of the ingredients.
10. When you have your desired flavor, pour the smoothie into a glass and serve with a straw.

<u>Ashwagandha Coconut Smoothie</u>

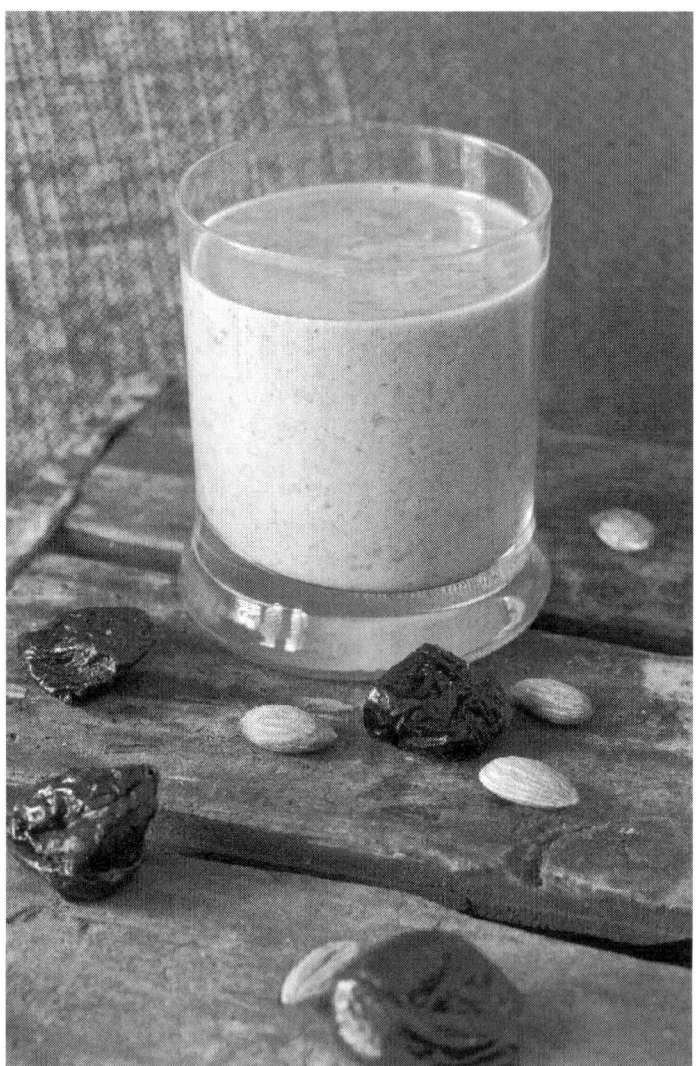

Serves 1-2

<u>Ingredients</u>

- 1 teaspoon of Ashwagandha powder
- ½ coconut milk
- 1 frozen banana

- 1 apple
- 3 dates
- ½ cup of blue berries
- ½ teaspoon of lime juice

Directions

1. Warm up the coconut milk in a stainless steel pan on a medium heat.
2. Add the Ashwagandha powder to the warm milk and stir while it is on a low heat.
3. Put the mixture in the refrigerator to cool.
4. You can make the Ashwagandha and coconut mix the night before.
5. Peel the apple and remove the stem and core.
6. Remove the pits from the dates and put the dates in the blender.
7. Add also the lime and apple meat.
8. Mix all the ingredients on a low to medium speed.
9. Mix them well so that all the flavors mix together.
10. Try the smoothie and add a little of one or more ingredients if it needs it.
11. When the smoothie is ready pour the smoothie into a glass with a straw.

Grape Smoothie

Serves 1-2

Ingredients

- 1 cup of seedless grapes
- 1 pear
- ½ cup of cranberry juice
- ½ cup of broccoli

Directions

1. Put the grapes into the blender.
2. Take the skin off of the pear and take out the core and the stem.
3. Put the pear meat into the blender along with the cranberry juice.
4. Cook the broccoli just until soft, then cool the broccoli in the refrigerator.
5. Put the broccoli in the blender with the other ingredients.
6. Put the speed on low to medium and mix together the ingredients until they are well blended.
7. Try the smoothie and add a small amount of one or more of the ingredients.
8. When the smoothie is ready pour the well-blended mix in a glass and serve with a straw.

Cucumber Beet Smoothie

Serves 1-2

Ingredients

- ¾ cup of cucumber
- ½ cup of beets
- 1/2 cup of hemp milk
- ½ cup arugula
- ½ teaspoon of lime
- Dash of salt

Directions

1. Peel the skin off the outside of the cucumber.
2. Cut up the cucumber, measure and put the cucumber in the blender.
3. Cut up the beets and put the beets in the blender.
4. Pour the hemp milk in the mix.
5. Cut up arugula and put in the blender.
6. Squeeze a lime and put the ½ a teaspoon in the mix.
7. Add the dash of salt.
8. Mix all the ingredients in the blender on low to medium.
9. Blend until all the ingredients are smoother than a puree.
10. Taste and add one or more of the ingredients if you need the change.
11. Once you get the flavor you desire pour the smoothie into a glass and serve with a straw.

Celery Green Smoothie

Serves 1-2

Ingredients

- ½ cup of celery
- ½ cup of broccoli
- ½ cup of carrot juice
- 1/2 cup of unsweetened apple juice
- ¼ teaspoon olive oil
- Dash of salt
- ½ teaspoon apple cider vinegar
- 1 teaspoon of chia seeds

Directions

1. Cut the celery into four sections.
2. Cook the broccoli just until it is soft.
3. Either buy a carrot juice from the refrigerated section in the produce section of the grocery store or juice ½ lbs. of carrots.
4. Pour carrots juice into the mixture.
5. Buy unsweetened not from concentrate apple juice, apple cider is great too.
6. Pour the apple juice into the blender.
7. Add the olive oil, salt, vinegar, and chia seeds.
8. Mix together the ingredients on a low to medium speed until everything well mixed together.
9. Taste your smoothie and if you need to add a little of one or more of the ingredients feel free to do so.
10. Once you get the flavor you want, serve the smoothie in a glass with a straw.

Lime Smoothie

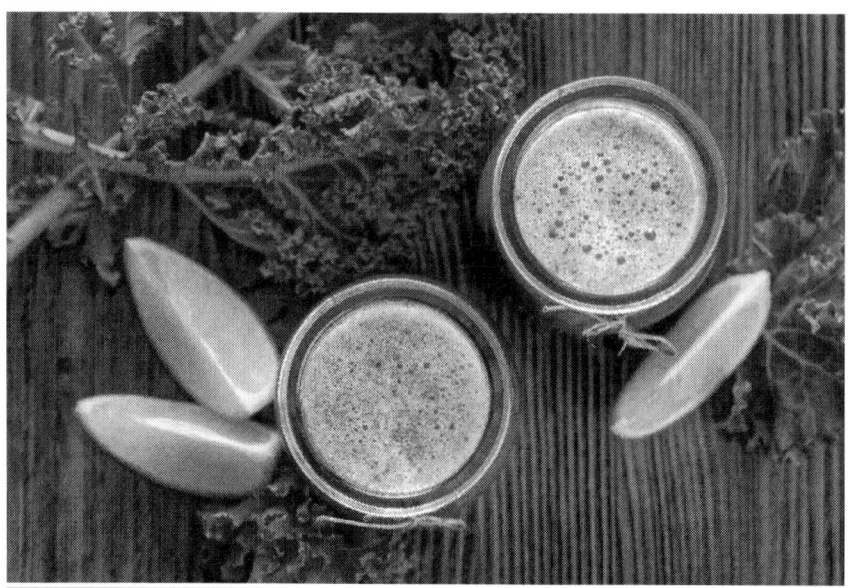

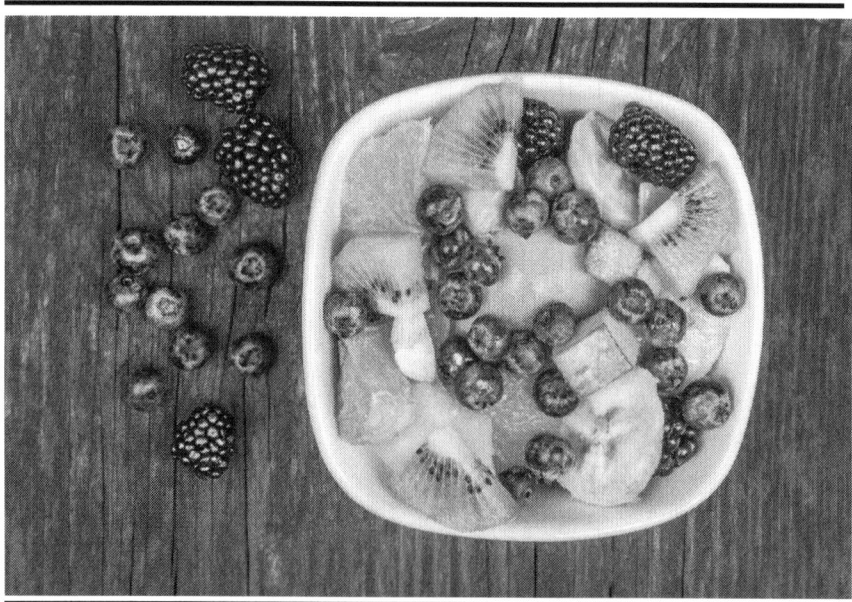

Serves 1-2

Ingredients

- ½ cup of celery
- 2 tablespoons of lime
- 1 tablespoon of lemon
- ½ cup of crushed ice
- 1/2 teaspoon chlorophyll
- ½ cup of kale
- ¼ cup of apple juice

Directions

1. Wash the celery and cut up the stalk to make the ½ a cup.
2. Cut the lime in half and squeeze the juice out to measure.
3. You might have to buy two limes to come up with the two tablespoons.
4. Cut the lemon in half to measure out the one tablespoon.
5. Put the celery, lime juice, and lemon juice into the blender.
6. Pour the crush ice into the blender.
7. Pull the leaves of kale off of the kale stems and put the kale into the blender as well. Pour the apple juice into the mix.
8. Mix all of the ingredients in the blender on a low to medium speed until everything is well blended.
9. Taste the smoothie and add a little of one or more ingredients if you think it needs it. Once you like the taste, pour in a glass and serve with a straw.

Arugula Smoothie

Serves 1-2

Ingredients

- ½ cup of arugula
- ½ cup of kale
- ½ cup of peaches
- ½ cup of almond milk
- ¼ cup of crushed ice
- 1 date

Directions

1. Wash the arugula and cut it up to measure.
2. Pull the leaves of the kale away from any stems and measure.
3. Cut a peach in half and take out the pit.
4. Take the date and cut the pit out.
5. Pour the ½ cup of almond milk into the blender.
6. Put the arugula, kale and peaches into the blender.
7. Add the crushed ice and date to the blender.
8. Mix all the ingredients on a low to medium speed.
9. Mix the ingredients well until they are pureed and the ingredients are smooth.
10. Pour a serving into a glass and serve with a straw.

Ayurvedic Pitta Avocado and Coconut Smoothie (Relaxing)

Serves 1-2

Ingredients

- ½ cup of avocado
- ½ cup of coconut
- ½ cup of almond milk
- ½ teaspoon of vanilla

Directions

Ayurvedic Pitta is warm to hot and oily in nature so to keep a happy Pitta stomach and system you want foods that are cool and on "the dry side" (in other words; foods that help you cool down your mind, body and temper).

The ingredients in the Pitta Smoothie are researched and approved for the pitta system. Take the avocado and cut the avocado in half and take out the pit.

1. Peel the skin from the outside of the avocado.
2. Put the avocado in the blender.
3. Either buy coconut in a package that has no added ingredients like sugar or sulfur dioxide.
4. If you cannot find dry coconut, you can usually find some in the freezer section.
5. You can also buy a fresh coconut and crack it open with a hammer and screwdriver.
6. Be very careful of course.
7. Poke a hole with the screwdriver and pour out the coconut water in a glass.
8. Strain the water with a strainer.
9. Set the coconut water aside for another smoothie or if you if you need more liquid for this smoothie you can use the coconut water.

10. Place the screwdriver on the side and tap the screwdriver with the hammer until the coconut cracks.
11. When you get a little bit of shell off you, you can then use a butter knife to help get the shell off.
12. Cut the brown skin off of the coconut meat.
13. Cut up enough coconut to measure.
14. Put the almond milk in the blender.
15. Take the vanilla bean and flatten it with your fingers.
16. Then take a knife and cut the vanilla bean longwise.
17. Scoop out the vanilla with a spoon to measure.
18. Mix all the ingredients in the blender on low and then mix on medium.
19. Make sure all the ingredients are thoroughly mixed.
20. When everything is mixed well test a little to see if it tastes good.
21. You can then add more of the ingredients to your liking and texture.
22. When you get the smoothie how you like it, then serve in a glass with a straw.

Ayurvedic Vata Berry Almond Smoothie (Balance, Focus & Relaxation)

Serves 1-2

Ingredients

- ½ cup of blueberries
- ¼ cup of raspberries
- 2 dates
- ¼ cup of watercress
- ½ cup of almond milk

Directions

In Ayurveda, Vata types are known for being cool, dry, and rough and they need foods that are oily, warm, and moist. The foods in this Vata smoothie are tested and approved for the Vata system. They help restore energy and balance- for the mind and body. They help vata's focus better without getting overstimulated.

1. Put both the blueberries and raspberries in the freezer the night before you want to make the smoothie.
2. Make sure you put the berries in a freezer safe container.
3. Pour the almond milk in the blender.
4. Cut the pit out of the dates.
5. Put the dates in the blender.
6. Wash the watercress and measure and put the watercress in the blender.
7. Put both the blueberries and the raspberries in the blender.
8. Mix all the ingredients together in the blender on a low to medium speed.
9. Mix them well and then taste a little of the smoothie.
10. If you want the smoothie thicker add more berries and if you want it thinner add more milk.

11. When you have the desired consistency and taste pout in a glass and serve with a straw.

Kapha Apricot Fig Smoothie

Serves 1-2

Ingredients

- ½ cup of fresh apricots
- 1/4 cup of figs
- ½ cup of fresh vanilla dairy-free vegan yogurt
- ½ cup of cabbage
- ¼ cup of cranberry juice

Directions

In Ayurveda, Kapha is consistent with cool, heavy, and oily so Kapha needs foods that are warm and dry for a nice balancing effect to get more energy for life.

1. Measure out the apricots and put in the blender.
2. Pour the cranberry juice in the blender.
3. Cut up and measure the figs.
4. Add the figs and the vanilla yogurt to the blender.
5. Cut up the cabbage and measure.
6. Put cabbage into the blender as well.
7. Put the cover on the blender and mix on low to medium speed.
8. When the ingredients are well mixed together then taste a little bit and see if you like the consistency and taste.
9. You can thicken with more yogurt or cabbage and thin out with more juice.
10. Once you like the flavor, serve in a glass with a straw.

Hemp Oil Smoothie

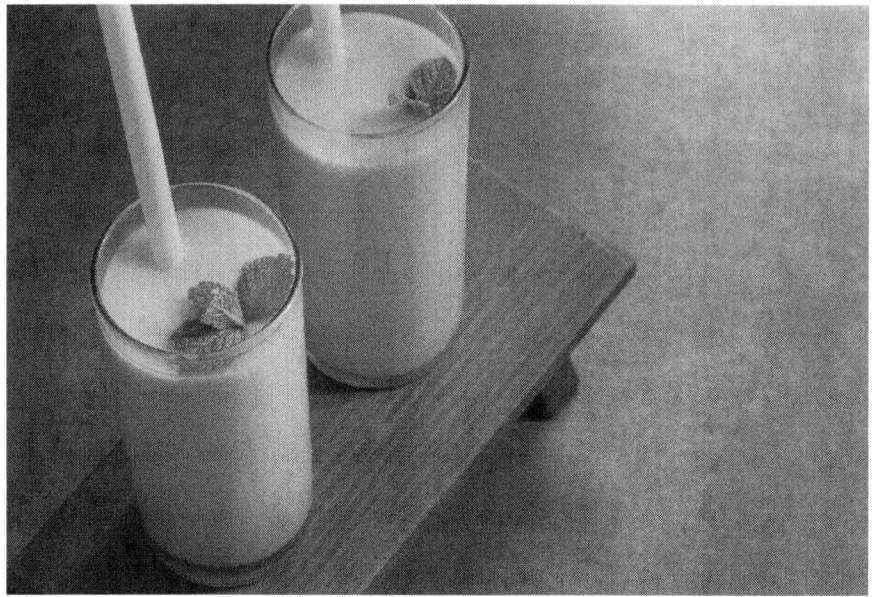

Serves 1-2

Ingredients

- 1 tablespoon of hemp oil
- ½ cup of almond milk
- ½ cup of apricots
- ½ cup of carrot juice
- ¼ cup of peaches

Directions

1. Buy carrot juice in the store or if you have a juicer juice ½ lbs. of carrots.
2. Pour the carrot juice in the blender.
3. Also pour the almond milk in the blender along with the hemp oil.
4. Cut up a peach and take the pit out.
5. Also cut up the apricot and take the pit out. Put both fruits into the blender.

6. Blend all the ingredients on a low to medium speed until they are well blended.
7. Taste the smoothie and add one or more of the ingredients if you think it needs it.
8. Once the smoothie tastes the way you want, pour the smoothie into a glass and serve with a drinking straw.

Cherry Mint Smoothie

Serves 1-2

Ingredients

- 3/4 cup of cherries
- 1 teaspoon of mint
- 1/2 cup of almond milk
- ½ cup of kale
- 1/2 teaspoon of fresh vanilla

Directions

1. Wash and cut the cherries.
2. Take the pits out of the cherries.
3. Put cherries into the blender.
4. Pour the almond milk into the blender.
5. Wash the mint and put the two sprigs in the blender.
6. Separate the leaves of kale from the stems.
7. Put the kale into the blender.
8. Press the vanilla bean with your hand and then cut longwise with a knife.
9. With a spoon, scoop out the desired amount of vanilla and put into the blender.
10. Blend all the ingredients together until smooth.
11. Taste your smoothie and if it needs a small amount of one or more of the ingredients then add.
12. When the smoothie tastes to your liking then pour into a glass and serve with a straw.

Coconut Oil Smoothie

Serves 1-2

Ingredients

- 1 tablespoon coconut oil
- ½ cup of cashew milk
- 1 frozen banana
- ½ cup of grapes
- 2 tablespoons Flax seeds

Directions

1. Peel the banana and cut it in half.
2. Put the cut banana in a freezer safe container and freeze overnight.
3. When you are ready to make the smoothie pour the cashew milk in the blender.
4. Put the flax seed in the coffee grinder and make a powder of the flax seeds.
5. Put the frozen banana, grapes, coconut oil, and flax seed powder in the blender.
6. Blend all the ingredients on a low to medium speed.
7. Mix the ingredients until they are smooth.
8. Taste the smoothie and if needs a little extra of one of the ingredients add to the smoothie and remix.
9. When you are happy with the flavor and texture of the smoothie, pour the smoothie in a glass and serve with a straw.

Pea and Carrot Smoothie

Serves 1-2

Ingredients

- ½ cup of peas
- 1 pear
- 1 apple
- ½ cup of carrot juice

Directions

1. Cook the peas until they are soft.
2. Cool the peas in the refrigerator.
3. Wash the pear and cut it in half.
4. Cut away the stem and the core until you are only left with pear meat.
5. Cut up the pear and put the pear meat into the blender.
6. Cut up the apple and take the core and seeds out.
7. Put apple into the blender.
8. Pour the carrot juice into the blender.
9. Mix all the ingredients together until they are smooth.
10. Taste the mixture and if you need to add a little bit of one or more of the ingredients, then go for it.
11. Once you have your desired taste then pour the smoothie into a glass and serve with a straw.

Don't forget to download your free complimentary eBook.

It's waiting for you at:

www.bitly.com/karenfreegift

Download it now, before you forget.

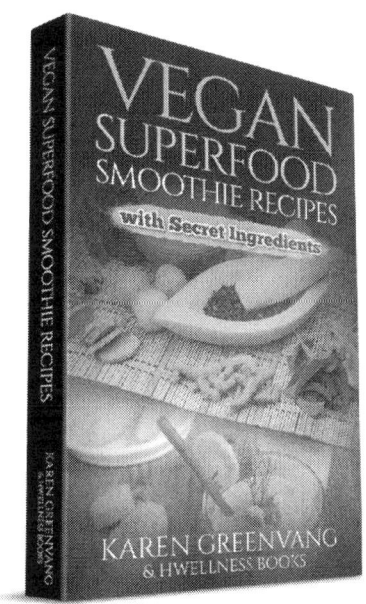

If you have any problems with your download, email me at: karenveganbooks@gmail.com

Conclusion

Making green smoothies is fun and exciting. It also makes a meal that is nutritious, easy to prepare, drink, and clean-up. We all need to save time these days. Making smoothies is also a very quick way to maintain and improve a healthy body. There are so many different combinations to try, you are bound to find three, four, or more you like and want to stick with for a long time. It is important to understand a few things when buying the ingredients for the smoothie. Should you buy organic or conventional fruits and vegetables? If you can afford to buy all organic food, it is in your best interest to do so. If you can afford to buy just some organic foods then buy the one that have the thinnest skin. A food like a banana has a thick skin that can keep out some harmful chemicals. So bananas you will be okay buying conventional.

Frozen over fresh food? It is a good idea to buy fresh foods. Food is always better fresh. The reason to put the food in the freezer for smoothie purposes is to get the smoothie cold. Adding ice to a smoothie can easily make it watery. Putting the food in the freezer before it goes in the blender makes the smoothie cold. There is generally nothing bad about frozen food, as long as it has not been in the freezer too long. Frozen food is a great way to protect food from spoiling.

You might want to know about canned food. Try to eat mostly fresh vegetables and fruits, but if you have to use canned food occasionally, it is fine. Sometimes you may have to use canned because of a seasonal fruit, or it just may be the only way to get a particular item for the smoothie.

It is possible that you may not like a smoothie at first. There is no hard rule about how a smoothie should be made so you can add or subtract any of the ingredients if you don't necessarily like something. Also adding to make your smoothie stronger is a supported situation, because everyone's taste buds are different.

The foods that make up these smoothies are healthy. Not everything good for you tastes good so sometimes you need to hide the flavor with another better flavor. This way you still get the benefits of the food you don't necessarily like, yet you do not have to taste it. You can always add but never take away so add a small amount of the ingredients after you have added the proper measurements.

I congratulate you for making a leap towards a healthy body. You will find that you may get sharper and even faster when you have been drinking these smoothies for about six months. You will start seeing a difference in your body and mind right away. Remember you can eat other things during the day as well. The smoothie is a great lighter meal or a quick energizing snack (for example before a workout) when the other meals you have can be a bit larger. Smoothies are light and easy meals that pack a world of nutrition in them. I hope you have enjoyed this smoothie book, and that some, if not all of the recipes are good for you. Thank you again for reading!

Karen

PS. If you enjoyed my book, it would be greatly appreciated if you left a review so others can receive the same benefits you have. Your review can help other people take this important step to take care of their health and inspire them to start a new chapter in their lives.

At the same time, <u>you can help me serve you and all my other readers</u> even more through my next vegan-friendly, holistic health recipe books that I am committed to writing.

I'd be thrilled to hear from you. I would love to know your favorite recipe(s).

Don't be shy, post a comment on Amazon!

> ➤ Questions about this book? Email me at:
>   karenveganbooks@gmail.com

Thank You for your time,

Love & Light,

Until next time-

Karen Greenvang

Book 2

Vegan Protein Smoothies

Superfood Vegan Smoothie Recipes for Vibrant Health, Muscle Building & Optimal Nutrition

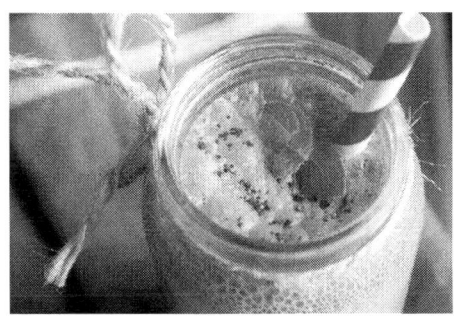

By Karen Greenvang (aka Karen Vegan)

Copyright ©Karen Greenvang 2016

www.HolisticWellnessBooks.com

Introduction

People who adopt a vegan lifestyle are often misjudged...

Often, you'll hear critics say things like, "How can you be vegan when you can't eat anything?"

But when living a vegan lifestyle, you can still enjoy a healthy, balanced and varied diet, with the ability to enjoy many different foods, meals and beverages.

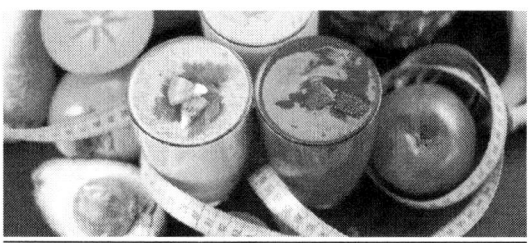

Most view the diet as being a response to animal cruelty and whilst this is a fantastic, motivating factor, another advantage of being vegan are the enormous health benefits it provides

Here are 5 benefits you'll experience from being vegan:

1. **Prevention of Cardiovascular Disease**

Studies have shown that adopting a vegan lifestyle can reduce the risk of type 2 diabetes and heart disease. By eliminating the unnatural dairy and meat products and eating more natural grains and nuts, people that adopt a vegan diet often experience increases in their cardiovascular health.

2. **Weight Loss & Increased Energy**

Natural weight loss is often a by-product of living a vegan lifestyle. A vegan diet eliminates most of the unhealthy, processed foods that contribute to weight gain and obesity. By avoiding foods high in saturated fat and sugar, whilst consuming healthier, natural foods like nuts, fruits & vegetables, vegans not only lose fat, but also experience an increase in energy. The avoidance is processed sugar is a big factor in a person's energy levels.

3. Avoiding Cow's Milk

Did you know that humans are the only species that continues to drink milk after childhood? Milk is not designed to be consumed into adult life and most adults are lactose intolerant or have milk allergies and don't know it. Vegan's drink healthier alternatives, such as almond milk or rice milk, which have added health benefits.

4. Eliminating the Risk of Salmonella & Mad Cow Disease

The deadly infection Salmonella, as well as Mad Cow Disease, are both illnesses brought on by eating animal products. The virus is usually contracted when a person comes into contact with raw eggs or raw chicken. Eliminating these foods from your diet means there is no risk of contracting the illnesses.

5. Healthy Skin & a Longer Life

The vitamins found in nuts and vegetables contribute to healthy and glowing skin. So, those who eat a vegan diet will experience an improvement in this area. Studies have also shown that vegans & vegetarians often live longer than those who are not. These benefits to health contribute to vegans having more energy, healthier skin, nails and hair and living longer by preventing major diseases.

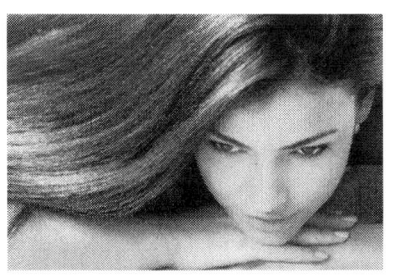

Amazing Vegan Smoothie Recipes That Are Naturally Rich in Protein

Peanut Butter & Banana Smoothie

This recipe contains two of the healthiest and tastiest ingredients you can use in a vegan Smoothie – peanut butter and bananas! The bananas are high in potassium, vitamin B6 and Vitamin C, while the peanut butter is an excellent source of protein. Infact, peanut butter is one of the best vegan sources of protein and should be featured in many of your vegan smoothies.

The bananas are best used frozen and I find the best way to freeze them for easy use is to cut them up into small slices, then spread them out on an oven tray with a sheet of baking paper on top. This way they will be easy to grab from the freezer and throw in the blender when you're ready to go! This smoothie tastes amazing and is packed with protein to give you an energy boost.

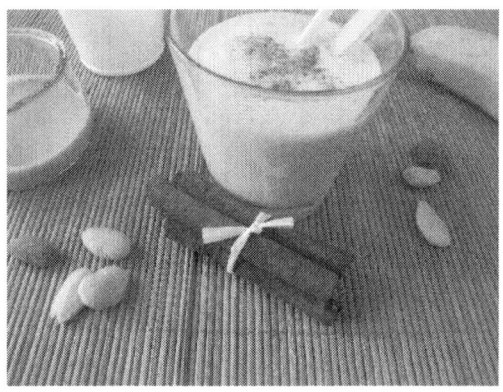

Serves: 1-2

Ingredients:

- 2 bananas, sliced
- 3 small pitted dates
- 1 heaped tbsp. of peanut butter
- ¾ cup of almond milk

Directions:

1. Place all ingredients in a high-power blender.
2. Blend until smooth and combined (if the mixture is too thick, you can add a small amount of water to thin out the mixture).
3. Serve into a chilled glass.

Almond, Flaxseed & Banana Smoothie

The banana makes yet another appearance, as it is a great fruit with amazing health benefits and great qualities for making a tasty, thick smoothie. Almonds are another great source of protein and are also low in saturated fats. Using almonds in this recipe as well as almond milk provides a healthy and high-protein shake.

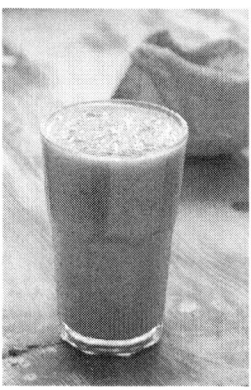

The flaxseed meal is an excellent source of Omega-3 fatty acids, aka 'good fats'. Good fats are also found in almonds, so this smoothie is packed full of both healthy fats and protein. After having this smoothie, not only will you feel full and satisfied but you will also get an energy boost from the banana's and natural source of protein. Peach makes it taste great!

Serves: 1-2

Ingredients:

- 2 bananas, sliced
- 15-20 almonds
- 1 big peach
- ¾ cup of almond milk,
- 2 tsp. of flaxseed meal

Directions:

1. Place all ingredients in a high-power blender.

2. Blend until combined and almonds are blitzed.
3. Serve into a chilled glass.

Tip: Add a small amount of water or coconut water (fantastic after workouts) if you want a thinner smoothie.

Blueberry Breakfast Smoothie

This blueberry breakfast smoothie is the perfect way to start your morning. It can be used as a meal replacement for your normal breakfast, as the ingredients used will provide you with enough nutrients and energy to keep you active and alert all day. If you're in a rush, sleep in or aren't usually a breakfast eater – then this smoothie will change your life! It's easy to prepare and will keep you going all day.

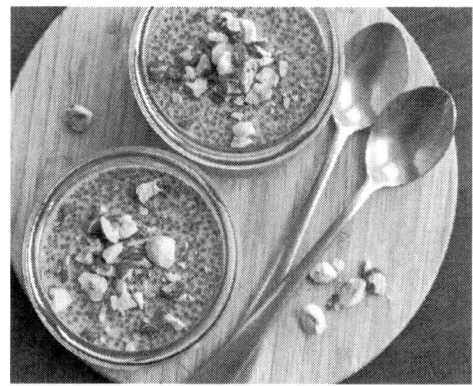

It provides a great slow release of energy from the oats, antioxidants and essential nutrients from the blueberries. It's thick, delicious and will make you feel full until your next meal.

Ingredients:

- 1 cup of almond milk
- ½ cup of fresh blueberries
- 2 tbsp. of gluten-free oats
- 1 tsp. of vanilla extract
- 1 tbsp. of hemp seeds
- 1 tbsp. chia seeds

Directions:

1. Add almond milk, oats, vanilla, hemp seeds and chia seeds to a high-powered blender.

2. Then, add the blueberries and blitz until well combined.
3. Pour into a chilled glass and serve. You can also use it to make a smoothie bowl- I love it before my workouts. Top it up with more nuts and seeds to create an amazing vegan energy breakfast!

Mango & Almond Butter Smoothie

It's no secret by now that nut butters are an excellent source of protein. Almond butter is high in protein, low in saturated fat and has a great taste. The almond butter gives this smoothie a thick, creamy texture making it taste amazing and is very filling. Mangoes are also a fantastic source of important vitamins that will help you stay energized and alert.

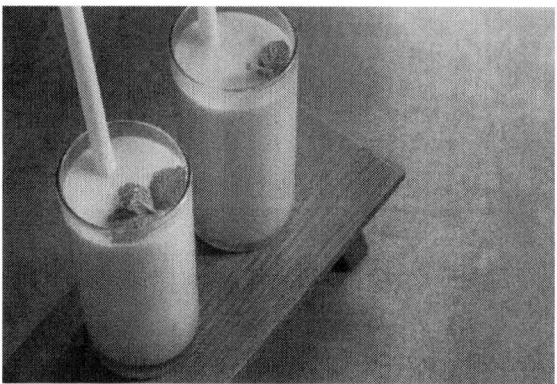

Try to avoid the bigger brands that are found in the spreads aisle and instead buy from an organic source in the health foods section. They cost a bit extra but it is definitely worth it.

This recipe also includes rice malt syrup, which is an alternative to maple syrup that is sourced from brown rice. It is a healthier option, as maple syrup often contains processed sugars, the rice malt syrup provides the same consistency and a similar flavour whilst also providing the health benefits of a complex carbohydrate.

Serves: 1-2

Ingredients:

- 2 cups of mango, cut into chunks
- ¼ cup of almond butter
- ½ cup of almond milk
- 1/3 cup of rice malt syrup
- A dash of water
- Mint leaves (optional)

Directions:

1. Add mango, almond butter, almond milk and rice malt syrup to a high-powered blender.
2. Blend together until well combined.
3. If needed, add a dash of water to thin the mixture.
4. Pour into a chilled glass, garnish with some mint leaves and serve.

Cinnamon & Apple Protein Smoothie

This is an incredibly delicious smoothie that can be used as a breakfast replacement if you are on the go. Cinnamon & apple is a classic flavour combination and when combined in this smoothie provides a great source of protein and vitamins. The main source of protein from this smoothie is from the oats and the almond butter. The apple provides a great hit of energy and the oats will provide enough protein and fibre to keep you full & satisfied as well as energies for the rest of the morning or afternoon.

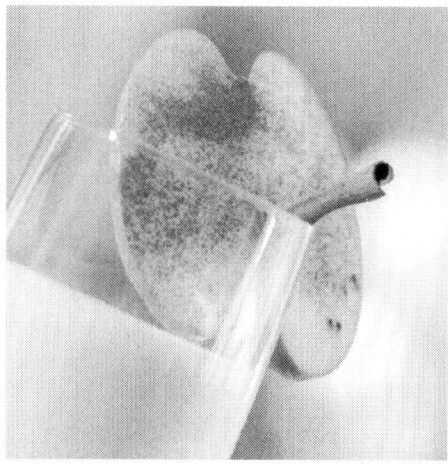

You can also use the apple peel in this recipe. The peel holds the greatest concentration of vitamins so it is a great benefit if you include it.

Serves: 1-2

Ingredients:

- 1 apple, sliced
- ½ cup of gluten-free oats
- ½ tsp. of cinnamon
- 1 tbsp. of almond butter
- ½ cup of almond milk
- A dash of water

Directions:

1. Add the almond milk and oats to a high-powered blender.
2. Pulse until well combined. Allow to rest for 2-3 minutes.
3. Add the rest of the ingredients to the blender and blitz until well combined.
4. Pour into a chilled glass and serve.

Spinach & Avocado Smoothie

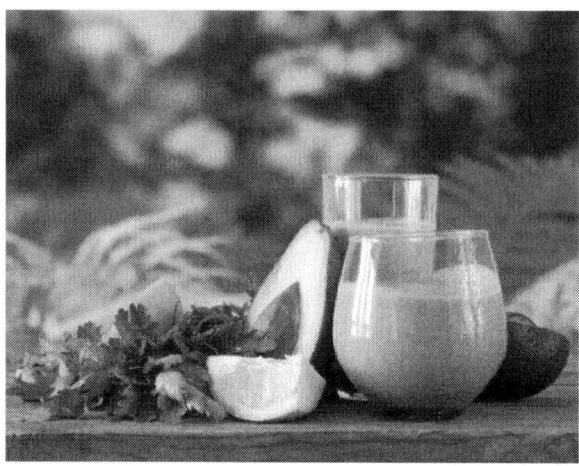

This savoury smoothie recipe packs its secret punch of protein from hulled hemp seeds. Hulled hemp seeds can be purchased in the healthy foods section of your local super market and are an incredible natural source of protein. Spinach is also a great all-rounder in smoothie recipes, blends easy, proteins an extra bit of protein and doesn't affect the flavour of the beverage at all.

Avocado is also a great ingredient to use in smoothies and other vegan recipes. It is super high in healthy fats and can be used as a spread, in smoothies or in a salad. This is a great green smoothie recipe that can be drunk at any time of the day. It provides a boost of energy to help get you through the rest of the day.

Serves: 2

Ingredients:

- 1 cup almond milk
- 1 cup spinach leaves
- ½ cucumber, chopped
- 1 tbsp. of avocado
- 2 large pitted dates

Directions:

1. Add all ingredients to a high-powered blender.
2. Blitz until well combined.
3. Pour into a chilled glass and serve.

The Green Machine Protein Smoothie

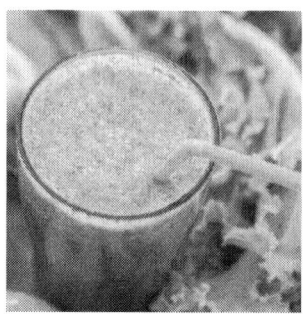

Here is an overview of all the greens you'll find in this vegan smoothie, along with the health benefits you'll gain from including them in your diet. The king of the greens found in this smoothie recipe is spinach. The hipsters of today are obsessed with Kale (don't get me wrong- I like kale as well) but spinach certainly rivals it and may even surpass it in terms of health benefits.

Spinach in packed full of iron (more than you will find in a T-bone steak) and has also been found to work as an appetite suppressant. If you drink this smoothie first thing in the morning, chances are you'll feel full for longer and it will help you lose weight!

Chard is packed full of anti-inflammatory antioxidants and studies have shown that it can help to prevent type 2 diabetes. This little known leafy green doesn't have the mainstream fame of kale or spinach, but including this vegetable in your diet will be a huge benefit to your health.

Water retention is a condition where the body holds more water than it should. The tissues absorb extra water and this can lead to complications and possible kidney disease, heart failure, lung disease and arthritis. The next two greens that are found in this recipe both help to prevent water retention, making them important players in this green machine smoothie!

Firstly, celery is a great source of fibre and B vitamins and will also contribute to the prevention of water retention. Cucumber is also packed full of fibre and B vitamins and will also join the fight against water retention. Cucumber is also a great source of electrolytes to give you a welcome energy boost.

Dubbed 'the beauty food', Watercress is the secret weapon in this green machine, protein-packed smoothie. Watercress is the leader of anti-aging vegetables, with enormous amounts of vitamin K and other healthy nutrients that contribute to healthy skin, hair and nails. If you want to look and feel younger, you need to start adding watercress to your diet and of course to your smoothies! Studies have also shown that watercress can help prevent cancer. Just another reason to add it to your smoothie every day!

Serves: 2

Ingredients:

- 1 cup spinach
- 1 cup cucumber, chopped
- ½ cup of celery, chopped
- ½ cup of fresh watercress
- 1 chard leaf
- ½ cup of almond milk

Directions:

1. Add all Ingredients to a high-powered blender and blitz until well combined.

Pumpkin Protein Smoothie

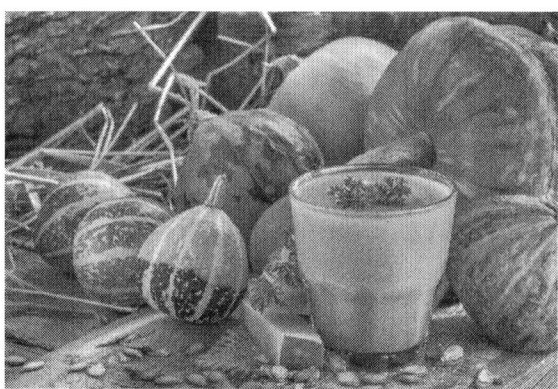

If you are looking from a break from the regular green vegan smoothies, this pumpkin smoothie is a great alternative. The pumpkin adds a filling flavour as well as a huge dose of vitamin A, which has a range of health benefits including healthier teeth, bones and blood cells.

The pumpkin protein smoothie is super easy to make and is a great option at any time of the day. Make sure you use an organic pumpkin puree to ensure it's the best quality and is vegan-friendly.

Serves: 1-2

Ingredients:

- 1 cup of almond milk
- ½ cup of organic pumpkin puree
- 1 tbsp. of organic almond butter
- ½ tsp. of cinnamon powder
- Small handful of hemp seeds, optional

Directions:

1. Add all ingredients to a high-powered blender.
2. Blitz until well combined.
3. Pour into a chilled glass and serve

The Ultimate Superfood Smoothie

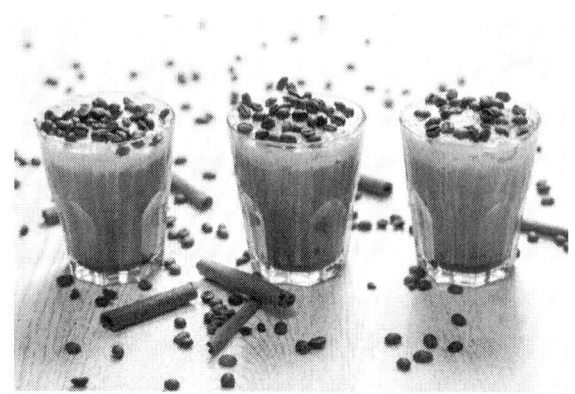

This superfood smoothie packs a protein punch as well as providing an array of benefits from the different superfoods used in the recipe. It will keep you energized for the most of the day and will help fight off those mid-morning cravings. Here is a list of the superfoods in this recipe, as well as the health benefits they provide:

Cacao Nibs – they are high in fibre, magnesium and iron. Magnesium is responsible for muscle and nerve function and help keeps hearth rhythm steady. Iron is necessary for red blood cell production and fibre is essential for healthy digestion. Cacao nibs are also a much healthier alternative to dark chocolate!

Maca Powder – is a root that belongs to the Radish family, and should be a popular superfood powder in every vegan's pantry. Maca powder is rich in vitamins B, C & E, as well as zinc, iron and magnesium. The antioxidants found in maca powder have also been shown to boost your mood, provide more energy and give you healthier skin.

Flaxseed Meal – This ingredient has featured in a previous recipe, and is very high in healthy omega-3 fatty acids. These good fats have been shown to have a positive impact on heart health and can help to prevent heart disease and cardiovascular disease. Packed full of antioxidants and fibre, some recent studies have shown the Flaxseed may help lower the risk of breast cancer, prostate cancer and colon cancer.

Chia Seeds – Chia seeds are another excellent source of healthy omega-3 fats. Another benefit of these healthy fats is that they raise HDL cholesterol levels, which is the good cholesterol that helps fight against heart and lung disease. They are also high in fibre, magnesium, vitamin B3, calcium, zinc and many other important nutrients.

Hemp Seeds – Hemp seeds are yet another excellent vegan source of healthy omega-3 fatty acids. What makes hemp seeds stand out from the others though, is the fact that it also boasts a good amount of protein. Adding hemp seeds to any smoothie is a great way to add an extra hit of protein to your drink.

Goji Berries – Goji berries contain a great amount of antioxidants that help to give you healthy skin and protect the eyes. They also help to boost your immune system. They also provide a source of complex carbohydrates which will ensure you have a sustained release of energy, helping you to keep active throughout the entire day.

Serves:1-2

Ingredients:

- 1 ½ cups of rice milk
- 1 banana
- 2 tbsp. of cacao nibs
- 1 tbsp. of maca powder
- 2 tsp. of flaxseed meal
- 1 tbsp. of chia seeds
- 1 tsp. of hemp seeds
- 1 tsp. of vanilla extract
- A small handful of goji berries, to garnish

Directions:

1. Add rice milk, banana, cacao nibs, maca powder, flaxseed meal, chia seeds, and hemp seeds into a high-powered blender.
2. Blitz until well combined.
3. Pour into a chilled glass.

4. Sprinkle Goji Berries or other fruits on top and serve.

Choc Strawberry Delight

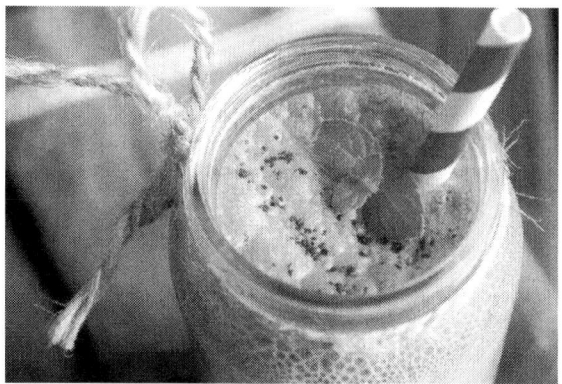

This chocolate and strawberry flavoured smoothie not only tastes amazing, but it provides a huge range of health benefits thanks to the superfoods that are included in the recipe. Strawberries have a huge range of healthy nutrients and vitamins including magnesium, phosphorus, potassium, iodine, folate, dietary fibre, vitamin B6, biotin and omega-3 fatty acids.

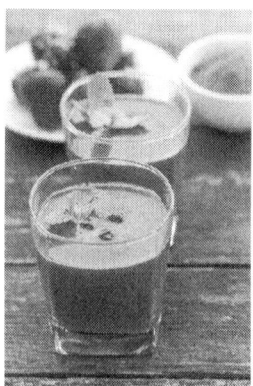

They are an excellent option for your smoothie and your vegan diet in general, as the health benefits they provide are incredible.

Serves: 2

Ingredients:

- 1 cup of coconut milk
- 1 cup of organic strawberries
- 1 tbsp. of cacao nibs
- 1 tbsp. of hemp seeds
- 1 tbsp. of chia seeds
- A small handful of raw almonds

Directions:

1. Add all ingredients into a high-powered blender.
2. Blitz until well combined and Ice Cubes are dissolved.
3. Pour into a chilled glass and serve.

Chia & Coconut Smoothie

If you aren't a fan of almond milk or you just want to mix things up, then coconut milk is another great option for a dairy free, vegan-friendly milk source. Coconuts are an excellent source of B vitamins, as well as A & E, iron, magnesium, calcium and sodium.

Chia seeds will give you a boost of energy and provide you with essential omega-3 fatty acids, while the protein source will be provided by the tofu.

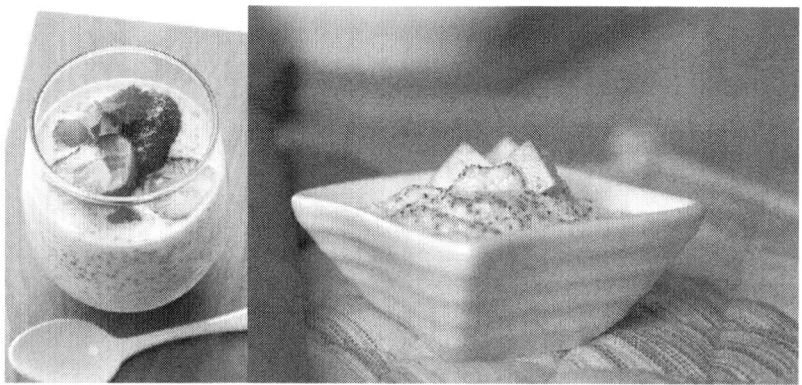

Tofu is one of the best sources you can find for protein that is vegan-friendly and this smoothie is a fantastic, tasty and super easy recipe for when you want a quick energy hit.

Serves: 1-2

Ingredients:

- 1 cup of coconut milk
- 4 tbsp. desiccated coconut
- ½ cup of water
- ½ of a banana, sliced
- 1 tbsp. chia seeds
- ¼ cup tofu
- Some fruits (for example strawberries to garnish)

Directions:

1. Add all ingredients into a high-powered blender.
2. Blitz until well combined.
3. Pour into a chilled glass, garnish with fruits of your choice and serve.

Tip: If the smoothie is too thick, add a small amount of water to the mixture and blend until it has reached your desired consistency.

Mango & Pumpkin Seed Smoothie

Perfect for a hot summer's day. The mango is one of those fruits that instantly makes you think of summer. When summer rolls around and mangoes are in season, there's nothing better than enjoying one in the sun and coupled with pumpkin seeds, this smoothie will not only quench your thirst and cool you down, but it will give you a mood and energy boost and have you energized and excited for the rest of the sunny day! But if it is a hot day and you are looking for a delicious smoothie that isn't too filling but will cool you down, then pumpkin seeds are a great source of natural high protein.

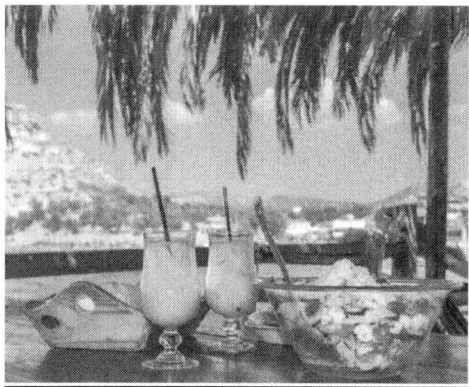

Serves: 1-2

Ingredients:

- 1 cup of coconut milk
- 1 cup of mango, cut into chunks
- 2 tbsp. of pumpkin seeds
- 1 tbsp. of coconut oil

Directions:

1. Add all ingredients to a high-powered blender.

2. Blitz until well combined.

3. Pour into a chilled glass and serve.

Protein Power Smoothie

We recommend using 2 tablespoons of sunflower seeds, but feel free to add an extra one if you really want a serious protein hit. This smoothie is great after a session at the gym, as it's a great way to help your muscles recovery quicker. The raw almonds are a great source of omega-3 fatty acids, and along with the banana, will help to replace some of that energy burnt off in the gym.

Ingredients:

- 1 cup of coconut milk
- 2 tbsp. of sunflower seeds
- 1 banana, sliced
- A small handful of raw almonds

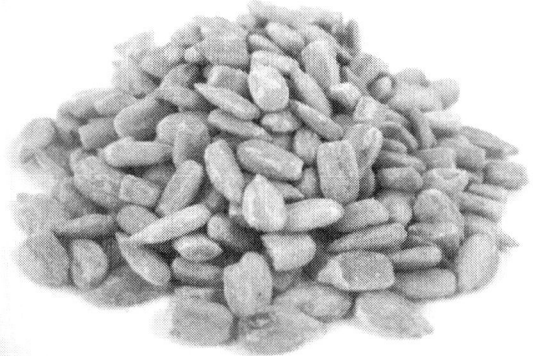

Directions:

1. Add all ingredients to a high-powered blender.
2. Blitz until well combined.
3. Pour into a chilled glass and serve.

Triple Chocolate Overload

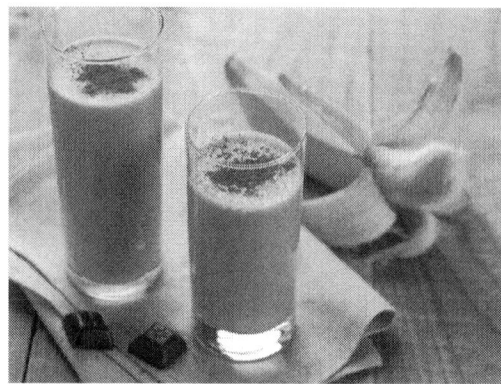

Chocolate lovers this is for you! And let's face it, who doesn't love indulging in chocolate? This recipe is appropriately named the 'Triple Chocolate Overload' as it gets its chocolate flavour from two different sources – Cacao nibs and cacao powder. The Banana and Almond Milk and there to provide a great consistency and a hit of energy, but let's not worry about that, because this one is all about the Chocolate!

Serves: 1-2

Ingredients:

- 1 cup of almond milk
- 1 banana, frozen and sliced
- 1 tbsp. of cacao nibs, or similar (for example raw, dark chocolate)
- 2 tsp. of cacao powder

Directions:

1. Add all ingredients into a high-powered blender.
2. Blend until well combined.
3. Pour into a chilled glass and serve.

Tip: If the smoothie is too thick, add a small amount of water to the mixture and blend until it has reached your desired consistency.

Blueberry, Vanilla Protein Smoothie

Blueberries are an excellent source of antioxidants, and are a great option for vegan friendly smoothies. They also pair excellently with coconut milk and almond butter, making this smoothie a healthy, flavoursome option for your repertoire. This is an excellent smoothie to have first thing in the morning, as the blueberries and almond Butter will give you a much needed energy boost to help you kick start your day.

If you are feeling adventurous, you can also add spinach or even oats to this recipe to make it even more flavoursome and healthier. The spinach doesn't affect the flavour at all and the oats will provide a source of complex carbohydrate for a sustained, long lasting energy release throughout the day. This smoothie is an excellent choice if you want to skip breakfast but still feel energized and full when you walk out the door ready to start your day!

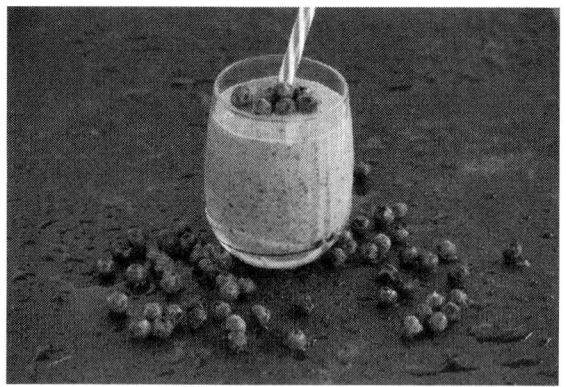

Serves: 1-2

Ingredients:

- 1 cup of coconut milk
- ½ cup of blueberries
- 1 tbsp. of almond butter
- 1 tbsp. vanilla powder
- 5 tbsp. organic oats, soaked in water

Directions:

1. Add all ingredients into a high-powered blender.
2. Blend until well combined.
3. Pour into a chilled glass and serve.

Trio of Nuts Smoothie

If you love nuts, then you'll go nuts for this smoothie. Nuts are nut butters are probably one of my favourite foods. They taste great, and the health benefits are almost endless. They provide a great source of healthy fats as well as being one of the best natural vegan sources of protein. They each have unique, delicious flavours, and when combined in the following recipe they taste amazing.

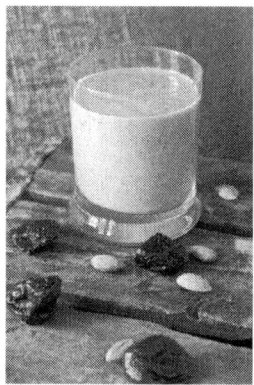

This smoothie is all about the nut. It uses three different types of nuts (almonds, walnuts and peanuts), and from three different sources (milk, butter and raw). It is an excellent treat to have post-dinner or just after lunch. If you want to change the consistency of the smoothie, try adding some extra water to make it thinner, or if you'd prefer a thicker smoothie, try adding an extra scoop of either nut Butter.

Serves: 2

Ingredients:

- 1 cup of almond milk
- ½ cup of water
- ½ cup of almond butter
- ½ cup of peanut butter
- A small handful of raw almonds
- A small handful of raw walnuts
- 1 banana, sliced and frozen

Directions:

1. Add all ingredients to a high-powered blender.
2. Blitz until well combined
3. Pour into a chilled glass and serve.

Tip: If the smoothie is too thick, add a small amount of water to the mixture and blend until it has reached your desired consistency.

Cashew & Spirulina Smoothie

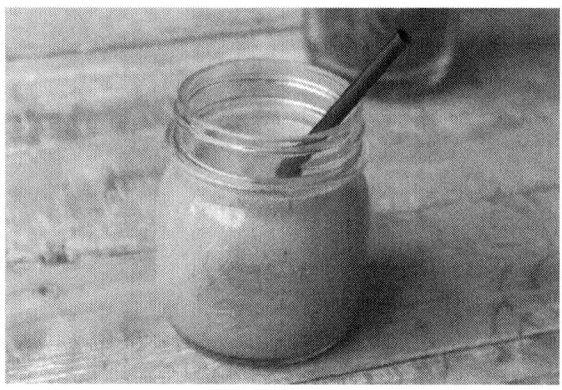

Another member of the nut family that is one of the best sources of protein is the cashew. Cashews are very rich and textured. They are delicious and I often find myself and handful after handful of cashews in between meals. They also work great in smoothies, cashew and cinnamon works great together.

Spirulina powder is another impressively beneficial member of the superfood family. It also boasts incredible health benefits such as vitamins B, C, D, E, A, potassium, copper, iron and calcium. I know a lot of people who absolutely love spirulina and swear by it, but I find that it can be a little bitter if you use too much. Therefore, I try to use it sparingly (as shown is this recipe), so that it doesn't over power the rest of the ingredients.

If you're not a big fan of spirulina, you can try replacing it with maca powder or hemp seeds. Using hemp seeds will give you an extra dose of protein for those post-work out smoothies.

Serves: 1-2

Ingredients:

- Handful of blueberries
- 1 cup of coconut milk
- ½ cup of raw cashews
- 1 tbsp. of spirulina powder
- 1 tsp. of cinnamon powder

Directions:

1. Add all ingredients to a high-powered blender.
2. Blitz until well combined.
3. Pour into a chilled glass and serve.

Peach & Oats Breakfast Smoothie

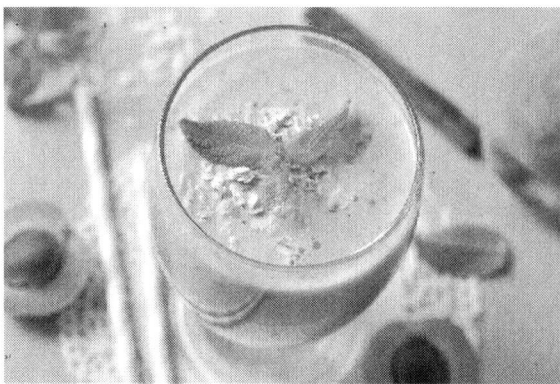

Who doesn't love the combination of peaches and oats in their morning breakfast? The peach is one of my all-time favourite fruits, it's absolutely delicious and goes tremendously well with oats in the morning. I would religiously eat peach & cooked oats for breakfast every morning, until I discovered this recipe. It uses the same ingredients (plus a few extras for added benefit) and gives you a big boost of energy in the morning. Not only that but it tastes even better than the morning oats I always use to have!

The fact that you can blend these amazing, healthy ingredients together and enjoy a delicious smoothie packed full of nutrients every morning is convenient and delightful. You'll also get yourself a great hit of protein thanks to the hemp seeds and rolled oats. If organic peaches are in season at your local super market, make the most of it and try out this fantastic morning recipe!

Serves: 1-2

Ingredients:

- 1-2 peaches, quartered with pits removed
- ¾ cup of almond milk
- ½ cup of rolled oats
- ½ cup of hemp seeds
- A dash of water, optional

Directions:

1. Add all ingredients to a high-powered blender.
2. Blitz until well combined.
3. Pour into a chilled glass and serve.

Cashew Butter & Oatmeal Morning Glory Smoothie

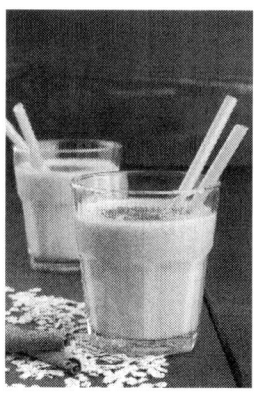

The title for this smoothie says it all. Once you've tried this recipe you'll literally bounce out of bed in anticipation ready to drink this incredibly delicious smoothie. Not only does it taste heavenly, but it is super packed with protein from the peanut butter and oatmeal. I've given it the name the 'morning glory smoothie' because I've found it to be such an effective mood booster, possibly due to the fact that peanut butter is one of my all-time favourites.

The hemp seeds are optional, I usually don't add hemp seeds, but if you're looking to get more protein into your diet then the watermelon seeds are a great way to do this. The morning glory smoothie will also provide complex carbohydrates from the oats, so you will get a sustained, slow release of energy throughout the morning. I'm often full of energy right through until lunch time when I drink this smoothie, with no cravings for snacks in between.

Serves: 1-2

Ingredients:

- 1 cup of rice milk
- ½ cup of cashew butter
- ½ cup of rolled oats (soak in rice milk overnight for a better result)

- 1 tbsp. of watermelon seeds, optional (for an extra protein hit)
- A dash of water, optional

Directions:

1. Add all ingredients to a high-powered blender.
2. Blitz until well combined.
3. Pour into a chilled glass and serve.

Leafy Green Dream

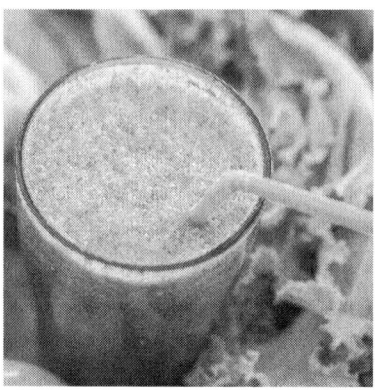

Those of you who can't get enough of your healthy leafy greens, this recipe is for you! Leafy greens are extremely healthy sources of beneficial nutrients and antioxidants. Including leafy greens in your diet helps to aid digestion and can help with energy levels by eradicating fatigue. If you are looking to add protein to your diet, leafy greens also play an important role as they help to metabolize protein in the body. Making the most of all the best leafy green sources, the leafy green dream smoothie will have you energized and fighting fit!

Serves: 1-2

Ingredients:

- 1 cup of almond milk
- ½ cucumber, chopped
- ½ cup of spinach leaves
- ½ cup of kale
- 2-3 leafs of chard
- 2-3 leafs of romaine lettuce

Directions:

1. Add all ingredients into a high-powered blender.
2. Blitz until well combined.

3. Pour into a chilled glass and serve.

Lime-Jalepeño Mango Protein Smoothie

Counting up the protein you get from the fruits as well as the hefty dose from the seeds, this smoothie packs a total of 14.5 grams of protein in this refreshing, sweet smoothie recipe with a spicy bite. If you're looking for a creamier texture and an addition of healthy fats, you can add half an avocado. That will add about 2 more grams of protein along with about 5 grams of fibre and a bucket load of potassium, as well as other nutrients, plus a smooth, mild flavour. You just can't go wrong by adding avocado to a smoothie! You can also serve it as a raw soup- season it with Himalaya salt and you're good to go!

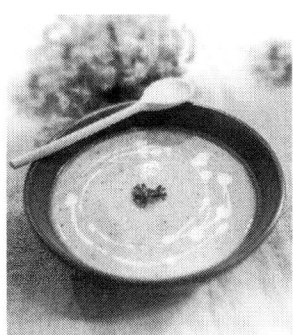

Serves: 1-2

Ingredients:

- 1 cup of coconut milk
- 1/2 lime, freshly squeezed
- 1 heaped tbsp. chopped jalepeño
- 1 tbsp. flaxseed, ground
- 2 tbsp. hemp seed, ground
- 1 tbsp. chia seeds, ground
- 1/2 avocado

Directions:

1. Add all ingredients into a high-powered blender.
2. Blitz until well combined.
3. Pour into a chilled glass and serve.

Tropical Mint Protein Smoothie

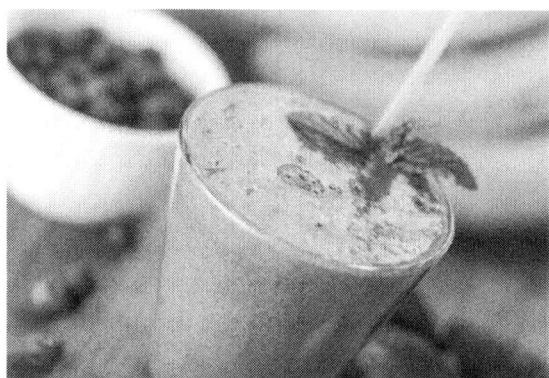

This is your all-day smoothie. If you have this filling meal for breakfast, you'll have energy the entire morning thanks to the fruit, and you won't want or need another meal until well into the afternoon thanks to the protein boost from the seeds. You'll get the nutrients but allow the wonderful fruit and mint flavours to help you feel refreshed all day. Acai berry puree packets are a great addition to keep handy and add to smoothies like these, but if you prefer just a simple mango, then that works great too.

Serves: 1-2

Ingredients:

- 1 large fresh orange
- ½ cup coconut milk
- 1/2 cups frozen mango
- 1 tbsp. ground flaxseeds
- 2 tbsp. ground hemp seeds
- 1 tbsp. ground chia seeds
- 4-5 fresh mint leaves
- 1 packet frozen Acai puree (optional)

Directions:

1. Add all ingredients into a high-powered blender.
2. Blitz until well combined.
3. Pour into a chilled glass and serve.

Pumpkin Orange Cream Smoothie

Do you find yourself drudging through your work day? Maybe the 2pm energy crash is a bit too familiar? The orange juice will help to revitalize with its vitamin C content, the ginger will relieve any inflammation in the body and will act as an energizer...

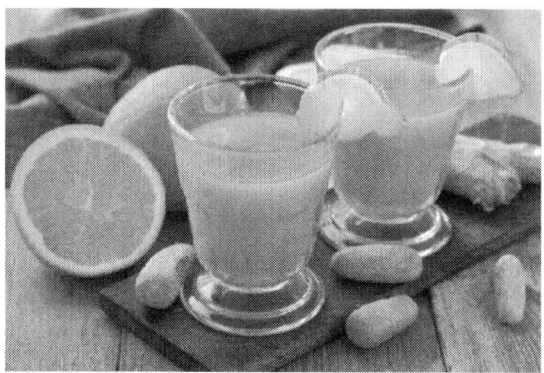

My favourite way to boost my spirits on a cold winter afternoon and sip on a healthy, refreshing drink.

Serves: 1-2

Ingredients:

- 1 medium orange, peeled and sliced
- 1/2 cup unsweetened orange juice
- A splash of vanilla extract
- 1/2 cup canned pumpkin puree
- 1/2 cup vanilla non-dairy yogurt
- 1 tbsp. maple syrup or stevia- optional
- 1 tbsp. grated ginger
- 1 tbsp. freshly ground flax seed
- 1/4 tsp. ground cinnamon

Directions:

1. Add all ingredients into a high-powered blender.
2. Blitz until well combined.
3. Pour into a chilled glass and serve.

Green Vegan Paleo Smoothie

This is a citrus and creamy wake me up smoothie, guaranteed to get you up and ready to go within seconds of drinking it. You'll get your daily boost of protein from the coconut cream and milk. Not to mention the sweetness from the mango and lime to give you that extra zing. The kiwi has an extremely high vitamin C content which will help fight any infections in the body and not to mention, spinach; a powerful superfood that will keep you young and glowing.

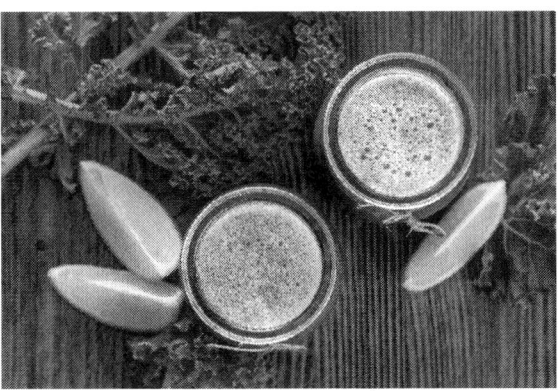

Serves: 1-2

Ingredients:

- 1 mango (diced)
- 2 cups kale (stems removed)
- 1 lime (juiced)
- 1 kiwi (diced)
- Handful of spinach
- 1 cup of coconut milk
- A dash of coconut cream (for extra thickness)
- Water

Directions:

1. Add all ingredients into a high-powered blender.
2. Blitz until well combined.
3. Pour into a chilled glass and serve.

Summer Fruits Quinoa Protein Smoothie

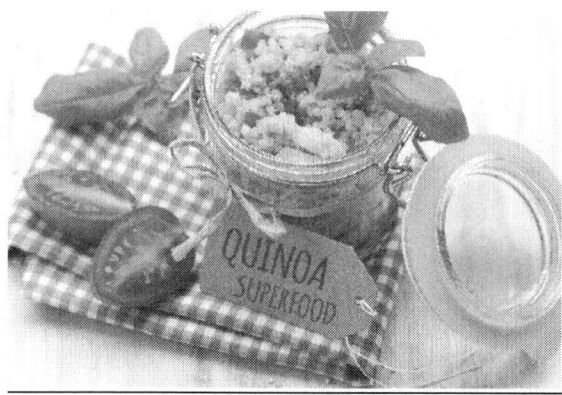

Did you know chia seeds contain some of the best Omega-3's found in plant form? In fact, chia seeds have more Omega-3 content than salmon, which is a true superfood.

Quinoa, another great source, is a complete protein, but it is also a prime source of magnesium, fibre and iron too. The ingredients go so well together with the mixed berries and thick coconut cream.

Serves: 1-2

Ingredients:

- 1-1/2 cups vanilla almond milk
- ¼ cup coconut cream
- 1/2 cup cooked quinoa, cooled
- 1 tbsp. chia seeds
- 1 tbsp. wheat germ
- 2 tbsp. maple syrup, stevia or other vegan sweetener-optional
- 2 cups frozen mixed berries

Directions:

1. Add all ingredients into a high-powered blender.
2. Blitz until well combined.
3. Pour into a chilled glass and serve.

Dark Chocolate Peppermint Protein Shake

Between the cocoa powder and the dark chocolate protein powder, chocolate lovers are going to want to drink this morning, noon and night. Which is absolutely fine, as dark chocolate contains a high amount of antioxidants and can help with stress regulation.

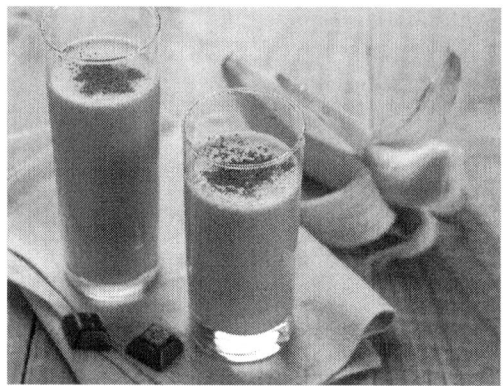

Soy sprouts powder is derived from natural plant sources and is very nutritious. This protein powder is very easily accessible and can be found in health food stores or online.

Serves: 1-2

Ingredients:

- 1 cup non-dairy milk of choice (I recommend chia seed milk for this one)
- 1 large banana, frozen
- 2 tbsp. dark cocoa powder
- 1 scoop soy sprouts powder
- 1/4 tsp. pure peppermint extract
- Pinch Himalayan sea salt

Directions:

1. Add all ingredients into a high-powered blender.
2. Blitz until well combined.
3. Pour into a chilled glass and serve.

Carrot Cake Protein Smoothie

For a dessert that won't undo a workout, blend almond milk, carrot juice, a banana, and sugar's healthy swap, cinnamon with a handful of cashews for a protein and vitamin E boost. Then sip. Aaaahh. And although it has the carrot cake flavour, it's much healthier than cake.

The cumin and cinnamon will give it that cakey taste, as well as providing you with the same benefits the Indians have been enjoying for centuries.

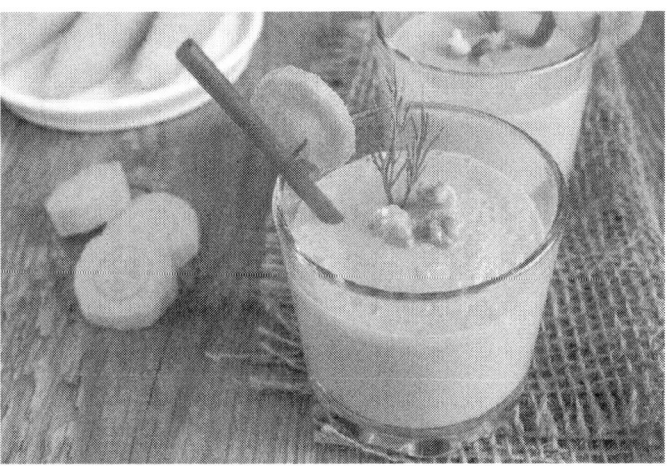

Serves: 1-2

Ingredients:

- ¾ cup vanilla almond milk
- ½ cup carrot juice
- 1 frozen banana
- Handful cashew nuts
- ⅛ tsp. cinnamon
- ⅛ tsp. cumin

Directions:

1. Add all ingredients into a high-powered blender.
2. Blitz until well combined.
3. Pour into a chilled glass and serve.

Caramel Vanilla Bean Hazelnut Milk

Luxurious, rich and absolutely splurge-worthy, this is a homemade hazelnut milk that is fit for a coffee shop and can be a great addition to your cappuccinos or black teas. This recipe uses a mix of soaked almonds and hazelnuts, but you can use just hazelnuts if you prefer. The flavour is caramelized with the addition of the Medjool dates, whole vanilla bean and cinnamon and you can turn it into a chocolate hazelnut milk quite easily by adding some organic dark cocoa powder. The possibilities are endless...

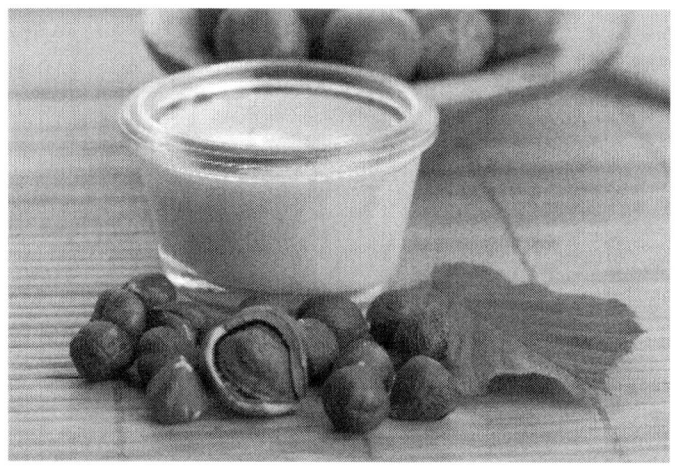

Serves: 1-2

Ingredients:

- 1 vanilla bean, roughly chopped
- 1/4 cup raw almonds
- 3/4 cup raw hazelnuts
- Halved 3 pitted Medjool dates, to taste
- 3 1/2 cups water
- 1/2 teaspoon cinnamon
- Pinch Himalayan salt

Directions:

1. Place hazelnuts and almonds in a bowl and cover with water. It's better to soak them overnight but you can get away with 1-2 hours.
2. Rinse and drain the soaked almonds and hazelnuts. Place nuts into a blender along with vanilla bean, pitted dates, water, cinnamon and salt.
3. Cover and blend for about a minute or until smooth
4. Place a nut milk bag (or a water separator bag) over a large bowl and slowly pour the blended mixture into the bag and gently squeeze the bottom to release the milk. Patience is key here. In the end you should be left with about 1 cup of pulp in the bag.
5. Rinse out blender and pour the milk back in. Now, pour it easily into a Mason jar and secure with lid. Chill in the fridge. Give the jar a good shake before drinking.
6. There are many ways you can use this smoothie, you can either drink it on its own, use it in cereals or add it to your oatmeal breakfast and as a creamer for your teas or coffees.

Conclusion

Thank you for reading!

I hope that with so many vegan-friendly recipes you will be motivated and inspired to start your journey towards meaningful veganism, vibrant health and total wellbeing.

Remember, the beauty of incorporating nutritious vegan foods into your daily diet is that you are making simple, yet sustainable changes that will work for your wellness long-term. Not to mention your spiritual wellness and taking care of the environment.

If you enjoyed my book, it would be greatly appreciated if you left a review so others can receive the same benefits you have. Your review can help other people take this important step to take care of their health and inspire them to start a new chapter in their lives.

At the same time, you can help me serve you and all my other readers even more through my next vegan-friendly recipe books that I am committed to publishing on a regular basis.

I'd be thrilled to hear from you. I would love to know your favorite recipe(s).

Don't be shy, post a comment on Amazon!

Thank You for your time,

Love & Light,

Until next time-

Karen Vegan Greenvang

Printed in Great Britain
by Amazon

45213660R00077